Say Goodbye To Overeating

A Non Diet Approach To Heal Your Relationship with Food

Monica E. Harris

Disclaimer: The content in this book, Say Goodbye to Overeating, is not intended to be a substitute for professional medical advice, diagnosis, or treatment. Always seek the advice of your physician or other qualified health provider with any questions you may have regarding a medical condition. Never disregard professional medical advice or delay in seeking it because of something you have read in this book. Reliance on any information found in this book is solely at your own risk. The author and publisher assume no responsibility for any outcome of the use of this book in self-treatment or under the care of a licensed doctor or physician.

While every precaution has been taken in the preparation of this book, the publisher assumes no responsibility for errors or omissions, or for damages resulting from the use of the information contained herein.

This book is for entertainment and informational purposes only. The views expressed are those of the author alone and should not be taken as expert instruction or commands. The reader is responsible for his or her own actions. Neither the author nor the publisher assumes any responsibility or liability whatsoever on behalf of the purchaser or reader of these materials. The reader is responsible for their own use of any products or methods mentioned in this publication.

This book includes information about products and equipment offered by third parties. As such, the author does not assume responsibility or liability for any third party products or opinions. Third party product manufacturers have not sanctioned this book, nor does the author receive any compensation from said manufacturers for sharing information regarding their products.

Table of Contents

Stop Binge Eating 101

How To Overcome Compulsive and Emotional Eating

Monica E. Harris

Introduction

I didn't want to stop overeating.

There. I said it.

Ice cream, pizza, potato chips, chocolate, any fried food... the list goes on and on. My favorite foods bring me a sense of comfort and, yes, sometimes, even joy. The actual problem is that I don't want to enjoy these foods in moderation. I want to keep eating until I can't eat anymore... and then I want to eat some more.

I have felt the shame of eating twice as much as everyone else at the dinner table. I've made promises to myself about dieting that have been broken as quickly as I could consume a box of double chocolate chip cookies. I've felt judgment from friends and family that criticize my eating choices. Many times, not because they want to hurt me, but rather because they love me.

This unhealthy habit is a real problem. Not only does it impact my health, but it hinders me from living my best life.

Maybe you can relate. And now that you understand a little about my struggle, you know you're not alone.

For me, something had to change. I couldn't see a future where life was different, but I knew I couldn't continue down this road. Not only did I change my life, but I am passionate about helping others overcome binge eating.

Overeating is not as uncommon as you may think. Research has shown that Binge Eating Disorder (BED) is treated in four out of ten individuals who are trying to lose weight.

So, are you struggling with binge eating or overeating?

Take a look at these signs and symptoms:
- You eat when you aren't hungry.
- You eat when you're full.
- Your eating habits feel out of control.
- You eat unusually large portions of food in a short amount of time.
- You feel embarrassed, guilty, or disgusted by your eating habits.
- You eat in secret or hide food that can be eaten at another time.
- You are continually dieting with no positive results.

If you identified with one or more of those statements, you are most likely somewhere on the overeating spectrum.

The good news is that this pattern can be broken and you can establish new habits that will enable you to begin living the life you've always wanted. You don't have to wait for something magical to happen that forces you to stop binge eating. It starts by simply choosing to change how you view food.

Now, before you stop reading because I've made changing your entire lifestyle sound far too easy, just wait. I don't want to trivialize how difficult it is to stop overeating. In fact, part of that choice may include reaching out for medical or psychological help, but self-help is a great place to start.

Having will power is not enough to fight off cravings that are so strong that they interrupt everything in your daily life. I realize that this change may result in emptying your pantry and refrigerator and making a clean start. But it's worth it to become a healthier version of yourself – you are worth it.

In the following pages, we will take a journey together. We will get to the root of when and how overeating became a part of your life. Then, we will explore how you can develop a new, healthy view of food. It won't happen overnight, and it won't be easy, but it's worth the sacrifice to live healthier and extend the length of your life.

In our present culture, overeating has often been trivialized as a lapse in judgment or poor lifestyle choices that result in eating too much. However, this disorder crosses gender and societal boundaries and has proven to be a much deeper issue. Those who struggle with perfectionism, high levels of anxiety, and social pressures find themselves at risk.

In 2003, the American Psychiatric Association (APA) recognized Binge Eating Disorder (BED) as a psychiatric disorder. This gave way for diagnosis and treatment for those who are suffering in a way like never before. It legitimized the seriousness of this disorder and those who suffer from it.

According to the National Institute of Health (NIH), Binge Eating Disorder (BED) is the most prevalent eating disorder, more common than anorexia and bulimia combined.

The Eating Disorder Foundation notes that BED is similar to anorexia and bulimia in how an individual needs to be in control. This is a constant internal struggle for those who overeat. When they binge eat, they recognize that once again, they have lost control. This can result in low self-esteem, depression, feelings of defeat and disgust, and distress. Some people are even impaired and crippled to the point they can't function in their everyday life.

However, when you learn to manage overeating, you begin the process of coping with your emotions, thoughts, and struggles with food.

So, if you are struggling with overeating, I promise that you will be in a better place by the end of this book. You will be equipped with tools that enable you to control what you eat and where food no longer controls you.

Today is the day you can choose to travel down a different path. You *can* establish new eating habits, and you *can* change the entire course of your life. However, if you decide to remain in the place you are right now, your overall mental and physical health will be at risk.

Those who struggle with binge eating often have problems at work, they avoid being around others, and generally have a poor quality of life. Typically, their physical complications include a laundry list of medical conditions such as heart disease, diabetes, joint problems, and more.

This book will offer helpful advice from leading eating disorder authorities. I will share my own story and what steps I have personally taken to become healthy. I'm a different person than I used to be. I've grown from painful experiences and have found healing in my mind and body as I've taken time to process the new me.

I believe you can also discover your path to a healthier and happier lifestyle. In the next chapter, we'll take the first step on this journey together.

Chapter 1: Identify the Root of Overeating

What Is Binge Eating/Overeating?

Overeating Versus Binge Eating

While many people use the terms synonymously, overeating and binge eating are not the same. There's a good deal of overlap in these ideas, and overeating *is* one component of binge eating, but those who overeat are *not necessarily* binge eaters. Moreover, binge eaters inevitably experience overeating. Overeating is a part of life, while binge eating is a serious and often debilitating condition. Know the differences between these two concepts to better understand your relationship with food and judge if your problem has risen to the level of binge eating. If it hasn't, you still need to be aware that overeating can quickly spiral into binge eating, so whoever you are, you need to ensure that you have a healthy relationship with food and that what you eat doesn't control how happy you are or take up hours of mental exertion. Too many people spend way too much energy thinking about what they're eating.

Overeating is a normal experience that all people face at one point or another. If you have bouts of overeating, be vigilant, but don't worry too much because part of enjoying food means overindulging occasionally. These episodes of overeating shouldn't give you feelings of immense guilt. If you've ever eaten cake at a birthday party even though you weren't hungry, that could be classified as overeating. When you stuff yourself full of food on holidays, that is also overeating, but in these cases, the frequency of overeating is low, and in healthy overeating scenarios, you don't beat yourself up over your actions. You're able to move on without letting that occasion warp how you behave in future food encounters. You go about your life without feeling self-hate and dread at your overeating.

Binge eating, meanwhile, includes overeating, but binge eating takes overeating to a whole new level and puts your head in an unhealthy space. You often subscribe to black and white thinking, and your actions become cyclical. Binge eating comes with feelings of distress as well as physical discomfort. When you binge, you feel ashamed and out of control. Plus, for binging, the rate in which you eat food is generally more rapid than normal. You don't enjoy the food. You are hurriedly eating it and trying to get as much into your body as quickly as possible. You may feel like an awful person for doing this, even though how you eat has nothing to do with your worth as a person.

If you noticed that your overeating has become more frequent and more compulsive, you might be wandering into binge eating territory. If your episodes of binge eating are happening at a high frequency, you may qualify for a full-blown Binge Eating disorder diagnosis.

Binge Eating Disorder

This is an eating disorder that is marked by eating enormous quantities of food in brief periods of time, leading to guilt, shame, bloating, fullness, and a feeling of losing your autonomy over food. For short, this disorder is known as BED. For a diagnosis, patients must have binge eating episodes for three months at a rate of at least one binge per week; however, even if you don't meet this standard, an eating disorder may be developing so don't take your binge eating lightly no matter how frequently you engage in behaviors. If you're binging only twice a month, that's still too many, and the information in this book can help you free yourself from food worry for good.

Out of all eating disorders, BED is the most common; it impacts three percent of women as well as two percent of men at any given time. Eight percent of people will have suffered this disorder within their lifetime. Further, it is the eating disorder that is frequently triggered by pregnancy and hormonal changes that are often normal parts of life. Whereas the onset of eating disorders often occurs in adolescence or young adulthood, binge eating can more often have onsets later in life and impacts both men and women.

While it is one of the most prevalent eating disorders, it often doesn't get the same attention that other eating disorders like anorexia nervosa or bulimia nervosa receive. It has only recently been included as its own diagnosis in the DSM-V, which is the guide psychological experts use to diagnosis patients with psychological disorders. Before 2013, BED was categorized under the now eliminated category of Eating Disorder Not Otherwise Specified (EDNOS), which was a grouping of disorders that didn't fall under the more specifically defined eating disorder categories. Luckily, with increased attention, BED finally got its own category in the DSM, but there's still ongoing work researchers need to do to understand more about this disorder.

Some common symptoms of binge eating disorder are as follows:

1. Fast-paced eating.
2. Consuming large quantities of food in a single sitting.
3. Being unable to control your eating.
4. Feeling stuffed to the point of discomfort.
5. Eating even when you aren't hungry.
6. Isolating yourself when you eat.
7. Being disgusted with yourself for your actions, or feeling anxious and depressed by those actions.

Binge eating disorder does not include compensatory behaviors such as purging. Using purging behaviors such as vomiting, laxatives, compulsive exercise, or fasting to alleviate the anxiety of binging fall under the category of bulimia nervosa.

Some side effects that you may have because of binging include other mental health disorders such as anxiety or depression, diseases like diabetes or heart disease; insomnia; joint pain; and menstrual irregularities. Binging wreaks havoc on your body and causes your hormones and regular functioning of your body to be erratic. Even your skin and hair may suffer from binging. Plus, one of the worst areas that binging influences is your digestive system. Binging may result in increased heartburn and acid reflux, IBS, diarrhea, constipation, and stomach pain. In some cases, one's stomach may even rupture from being so full, so the dangers of binging are very real, and you must take them seriously.

Unfortunately, while data says that nearly ten million Americans suffer from this disorder currently, BED is widely underdiagnosed, and many people who have it never seek treatment. Often, shame and stigma lead to people not wanting to come forward with their struggles, making it a disorder that has been under-researched and is shrouded with secrecy, but with some education and helpful tips, you can put an end to your binge eating forever. It may seem impossible to cut it out of your life, but people do get better, myself included.

How to Identify if Binging Is a Problem?

If you're reading this book, you probably already suspect that you or someone you love may have a problem with binge eating. Chances are that even if you do not binge frequently enough for a BED diagnosis, you may have a binge eating problem. The fact that you are concerned about your eating habits shows that you probably have that out of control feeling when it comes to food. Even if you just overeat, the advice in this book can show you how to keep a healthy relationship with food and ensure that your bad habits don't lead to you developing an eating disorder.

Even though you've picked up this book, you might be saying to yourself, "I don't think my problems are bad enough to be serious, but I want them to stop," and that's a common mentality to have. Many people think that their issues aren't severe enough to be serious or that they're making a big deal out of nothing. On the contrary, eating disorders and disordered eating are always serious.

Being that humans must eat, you cannot escape food. Thus, if your relationship with eating is dysfunctional, you'll never be able to experience the joy and peace of mind that you deserve.

For a long time, I didn't realize that my food behaviors were a problem because of biases I wrongly held and the teachings of a weight-loss driven society. I thought that my binges were a result of a lack of will power and didn't understand why I couldn't get my act together and get the extra pounds off. I have since learned that my behavior was perfectly logical. It wasn't healthy, but there was a name for what I was experiencing, and being able to use the word binge after having no language for what I was doing helped me change my life and kick binge eating aside for good. It's been nearly seven years since I've last had a binge when at one point, I couldn't even go three days without one!

The first step is acknowledging that your relationship with food is warped. Don't try to belittle your problems because food should never be the enemy. It keeps you alive and gives you the power to do amazing things. Without food, you would die, so it's time to stop feeling bad for eating. Even if you eat too much, that's better than not eating enough to sustain your body as long as you've accepted that you can't control your urges and need to coexist with them.

If you have had multiple experiences of ingesting food far past the point of being full and feeling out of control around food, you likely have some kind of eating disorder or, at the very least disordered eating. If you find yourself constantly thinking about your next meal or worrying that you'll lose control at a buffet, you have a problem. Whenever food starts to take up hours of your time each day, that's when you know you need to change. Eating should be instinctual and feel good. You shouldn't be stressing out over every meal. If you are, yet again, that's an indicator of a problem. Trust your gut on this. If it is telling you that something is wrong, something probably is! Let yourself accept the help that you need. Most importantly, know that you're not going through this journey alone.

You're Not Alone

I began binge eating in junior high, maybe even younger, but my issues worsened when I was eighteen in my second semester in college, feeling like the worst person alive. I'd always been an emotional eater, eating to cope with whatever I was feeling, ranging from anxiety to sadness to joy. I used food as both a reward and punishment, and in the process, my relationship with eating became twisted. I began to dread food, even though it was the part of my day I most looked forward to. I began hiding out in my room and munching on all the chips and sweets I could find. I'd gorge myself on anything just to fill the pit in my stomach that constantly seemed to be begging for salt and sugar.

I was an active child, so for a while, I was able to engage in these behaviors without gaining weight. I still felt guilty for what I was doing, but in high school, I began putting on weight at a rapid pace, and I started feeling increasingly worse about myself. The lower my self-esteem dropped, the harder it became to control what I was eating, so I kept putting on weight, which made me feel more unhappy and led to more binge eating to cope with the self-hate I felt! My self-hate was about more than my weight, but at the time, I thought that losing weight would make everything better. When I got to college, I was so dissatisfied with myself that I was desperate to make changes as quickly as possible, and this want led to me abusing my body and confusing it.

My final downward spiral started with a very simple pursuit that I'd seen friends and family members experience for years: a diet. Wanting to counteract the freshman fifteen, I vowed to lose weight, and I didn't realize all the negative impacts that weight loss could have on my mind and body. When I started binging more frequently despite my dieting efforts, I felt out of control— like a monster— and I had no idea how to make it better, so I lived with the shame and guilt that come with binging, and I didn't think that anything would ever change. By day I tried to lose weight, but by night, I became the ravenous binge monster. I isolated myself from my friends and spent my spare time being hungry no matter how much I'd already eaten. I was in a war with my hunger, and I wasted countless hours fighting with myself to try to find a semblance of control over my body, which kept doing things that I didn't want it to do.

I spent over a decade battling my hunger, and I never felt so hopeless as I did then. During my extreme binging years, I felt that my binge eating made me a freak and separated me from my peers. I self-isolated and became ashamed of my behaviors rather than reaching out and seeking change. My entire lifestyle suffered because of my twisted relationship with food. Yet, even in the height of immense dysfunction, it took me a long time to want to change. To change, I had to realize how common binge eating is and how our culture encourages this problem more than it tries to prevent it. I had to learn that my disorder wasn't because I was a bad person; it was because of my circumstances as well as a society that failed me. While eating disorders have biological roots, they also have deep societal roots. Thus, you are not alone with your binge eating, and you shouldn't feel like your binge eating reflects poorly on your character because it is a common problem that is created by a culture that fixates on unsustainable methods of weight loss.

Who Is Impacted by Binge Eating?

Binge eating impacts a wide range of people, so anyone can have it. People of all genders, races, and socioeconomic classes face this issue. Further, binge eating can occur among people of any size. It is most common for binge eating to occur in obese people. Those with a family history of binge eating will be more likely to binge eat, and childhood trauma can increase people's chances of developing BED. It is more common, but not significantly, among women than men. Among women, binge eating begins between the ages of eighteen and twenty-nine while among men, this disorder is often seen later in life between the ages of forty-five and fifty-nine.

As for socioeconomic factors, research has suggested that binge eating may be more dependent on income for women than for men, but cases were also seen across social classes. A Project Eat experiment suggested that those of higher socioeconomic status were more prone to binge eating when they were dissatisfied with their bodies, dieted, and were mocked about their weight by family members. These factors, however, were not as influential on people of lower socioeconomic status. For those of lower socioeconomic status, factors like being obese or overweight, dieting, and not having good access to food often led to binge eating.

Whatever your circumstances, you may be at risk for binge eating disorder if you have any signs of frequent emotional eating or an otherwise warped relationship with food. Likewise, if you have an obsession with your weight or diet, you may also develop a problem with binging. While a range of factors leads to binge eating such as food scarcity and access to addictive, less nutritious foods, one of the biggest contributors to binge eating is a diet culture that promises fast, easy weight loss results.

The Culture of Binging and Why Dieting Is Bad

Unfortunately, we live in a culture that is fixated on the number on the scale more than it is fixated on the health of people who are pushed into unneccessary diets. Perfectly healthy people start diets every day just because it seems like they should. A social emphasis is put on weight, and in the process, people become predisposed to dieting, which often leads to binge eating because of the unrealistic parameters that diets have. Therefore, to fix your binge eating problem, you need to understand how diet culture plays into your issues and how to resist the allure of diets. Contrary to what you may think, you cannot stop binge eating if you continue to diet. Once you stop binging, you will be able to make healthier choices and eat more foods that nourish you on your journey to freedom from binging. For now, don't restrict yourself at all. To stop binge eating, you must vow to never go on a diet again. It may seem hard to promise this because the idea that you may never lose weight is painful to countless people, but I was at my heaviest weight when I was at the height of my binge eating due to the neverending hunger that filled me. I did eventually lose weight, but as I stopped dieting, I noticed I didn't worry about it as much. I was happy in my skin after years of hating who I was.

For a long time, I thought that if I could just find the right diet then I could lose weight and start eating normally. But the more I tried to resist my need for food, the more I binged, and the more weight I gained. It was an endless cycle of trying to deprive myself, getting fed up, binging, and feeling shame. I discovered that you can't force your body to be a size it doesn't want to be. So don't dream of being the weight of a model on the cover of a magazine. First of all, she's probably been heavily photoshopped, but more importantly, one size does not fit all. What's healthy for one person may not be healthy for you. People have natural body weights based on factors like genetics, so you shouldn't compare yourself to others to determine your health.

Some theorists have come up with the idea of a set point weight that all people have, which is a weight that your body tends to maintain when you eat intuitively (which few people do because of our diet culture). The set point theory of weight suggests that based on genetic factors, your body wants to be a certain weight, which is the weight that will best keep you healthy based on your specific needs. Some people have a higher setpoint, while others have a much lower set point. It is also important to understand that people will have shifting set points throughout their lives. These changes won't be significant, but older people often gain weight because of metabolic changes that naturally occur. Your body tries to regulate your weight when it is left to its natural devices; thus, while having more weight isn't bad, many people may rise above their set point weight when they are binging, leading to them feeling uncomfortable in their skin and not feeling as energized as they should.

The set point theory comes down to your brain and your hormones, which function together to maintain balance in your body. Your hypothalamus is the part of your brain that is signaled by your fat cells. Your fat cells help your body determine your nutritional needs throughout the day. Hormones, like leptin that helps you feel satiated, and ghrelin, which makes you hungry, will be used by the body based on stimuli it receives and patterns from your daily activities. Naturally, your body lets you know when you need food and when you don't, but when you use a diet, your body's signals are thrown out of whack, which can result in weight gain. Set point theory suggests that when you restrict your food intake, your body will start to focus more on food and slow down your metabolism to maintain its weight.

While not all scientists believe in set point theory, it speaks to the idea that when you were born, your body knew when you were hungry. As a baby, you cried when you wanted food, instinctually knowing that you were hungry. Thus, there's a way to find peace with food now too. You just have to get the cacophony of diet culture out of your head to do so, which, given how many diet ads and unhealthily thin models you see daily, is hard.

Our eating habits are often a game for companies. While over forty-percent of adults are obese and the dieting industry continues to get larger, obesity rates are not leveling off, which shows that very little change is being produced by our diet culture. Rather, companies are exploiting body standards and pressures to make more money. They convince you that you're not happy with the way you are because of your weight. But when dieting doesn't help make you happier, they blame the failure on you being lazy and lacking willpower. The reality is, they are evoking the *exact* reaction that they want.

We live in a culture that glorifies many things that lead to dieting and shame around weight, but we never benefit from these glorifications. After all, they are used against us in advertising because those who cannot embody the glorification are then shamed into giving into unhealthy demands. Don't let these glorifications hurt you any more than they already have. Rise above them.

One of the most poignant glorifications is the glorification of thinness or having muscled bodies. Women tend to be convinced that they need to be thin while men usually are convinced that they need to be more muscular. Both are ideals that countless people can't feasibly reach. Over fifty percent of Americans feel dissatisfied with their current weight. Among women who are of a healthy weight, seventy percent want to be thinner. A stunning eight percent of ten-year-olds are afraid that they will be fat. By thirteen, over half of girls don't like their bodies, and by seventeen, that number goes up to seventy-eight percent.

Our culture glorifies overconsumption. In more than just food, academics such as Kima Cargill suggest that our culture of constantly wanting more leads to imaginative hedonism, which is the idea that we envision the triumphs that certain products can give us but are disappointed when those objects don't give us the happiness we expected. This same overconsumption is rooted in diet culture in interesting ways. While the food industry tries to sell us happiness with addictive foods, the diet industry works symbiotically selling us over consumptive methods to lose the weight binging has put on (or that we naturally have based on our set points).

Moreover, our culture glorifies dieting. Because of the latter two glorifications, the celebration of dieting means that we are unable to live up to the expectations of eating plentifully and being thin. You can't both overconsume and be stick thin, so people are forced to teeter between binging and dieting. With so much body satisfaction, diets start young. One-third of children aged ten to fourteen are on diets. Further, a third of teen boys and more than half of teen girls use dangerous methods to manage their weight, such as restricting their food intake, smoking, throwing up, and using weight loss drugs. Among nine to eleven-year-olds, a reported eighty-two percent of families identified as sometimes or very often engaged in active dieting. These numbers are startling and show the unhealthy Western fixation on dieting itself. Even people who don't need to be dieting are being convinced that it's a normal part of growing up. Not only do we binge on food, but we, as a society, binge on erroneous lies that have been spread about the correlation between weight and eating.

Ironically, our culture glorifies eating as much as it glorifies weight loss. As has been discussed, companies use food against us to make us eat more and to encourage overeating. The issue is not just that they are getting us to eat more, but they are encouraging us to consume foods that are addictive and unhealthy. We are inundated by commercials selling us hyper-palatable foods that can lead to addiction. The advertising targets children, especially, engraining over consumptive eating for the youngest of society. Ads highlighting bulk products for discounted prices and addictive foods contribute to the childhood obesity epidemic that is causing the weights of children to skyrocket and setting them up for a future of dieting. Research has shown that these ads predominantly highlight unhealthy foods. Children who watched over three hours of TV per day are more likely to be obese by fifty percent, showing the role of advertising in the glorification of overeating. People are taught that the more you eat, the better you will feel. This simply isn't true. Food ads link success with eating hyper-palatable foods, but in reality, the companies are trying to get you addicted so that you buy more.

The foods that are heavily advertised are full of simple carbs with lots of unhealthy processed sugar and trans fats. These foods are associated with health issues, and they give people spikes in energy and then crashes, which leads to people wanting more just to keep their energy levels up. Everyone can easily bring to mind a hyper child who has had too much sugar and then crashes shortly later. This same effect happens in adults too. We feel energized for a few hours, and revert back to being exhausted. Many experts suggest that sugar could have the same levels of addiction as opiates, since the processes that occur in the brain are markedly similar. Many people who binge eat may also have chemical dependencies, showing that bingers may have more addictive personalities. When we eat sugar, feel-good chemicals like dopamine are released, and our opiate receptors are opened. Thus, we become more compulsive with our eating and other behaviors. Sugar can lead to more headaches, and hormonal problems. We can also become chemically addicted to it, meaning that when we deprive ourselves of sugar, we may eventually binge on it to lessen the withdrawal symptoms and cravings.

The dieting industry promises us a cure to the problems posed by food companies. The dieting industry is a mammoth industry that is worth seventy-billion dollars as of 2019, which is an increase in revenue despite the growing resistance to dieting because of the body positive movement. Diet culture makes people insecure, while body positivity allows people to stop dieting altogether. No one needs to be on a diet. The bottom line is that the diet industry isn't trying to help you. It's there to keep you trapped.

Diet culture is created to hurt us by keeping us in a cycle of wanting and failing to lose weight. Diets don't work, so companies keep you going on and off diets, making you think that if you have enough willpower that maybe someday one of those diets will work. When you look at the statistics on dieting, it is startling to see how widely diets don't work. Researchers estimate that up to ninety-five percent of diets fail, and people generally regain lost weight within five years. Further, of the five percent who do lose weight successfully, ninety-eight percent match the clinical qualifications of having eating disorders. With this in mind, dieting doesn't do much good for anyone. Your options are to keep diet cycling, have an eating disorder, or make peace with food. I know which one I'd pick if I were in your shoes.

Food is representative of other problems in our lives, and companies know that. Often, we try to control our food as a way to deal with the hardships we sometimes face. I spent years thinking that my weight was the biggest problem in my life when it wasn't! The weight loss commercials not only suggest that using their product will result in weight loss, but also that your whole life will change as a result of losing weight. The truth is, though, your weight doesn't cause you to binge. You binge because of how you feel about yourself, which goes much deeper than your weight. When you feel insecure about your weight, you begin to question your worth as a person, which leads to your relationship with food, becoming even more detrimental to your well-being. Binging is not just about food; it's about your feelings and views of yourself too. Diet culture promises you happiness, but the only way to acquire happiness is to learn to love yourself as you are.

Restriction of food commonly leads to binging. The statistics don't lie. Young girls who go on diets are twelve times more apt to binge eat compared to those who don't diet. When you restrict food, not only does it throw off the chemical processes in your body, it makes your brain think that you are at risk. Your brain begins to worry that you are facing a famine and your body begins to slow down its metabolism to conserve energy. Afterall, your body is wired for survival, so when you try to lose weight, your body will fight you because it is trying to ensure that you stay alive. While famine for most people in the Western world isn't a predominant concern, your body is still used to times in the history of humanity in which famine was a pressing concern. Thus, diets force you to fight your very instincts.

The very way in which people are classified as either unhealthy or healthy shows the gross misunderstanding of how people's bodies work. It's important to realize, therefore, that there are several flaws in how people are classified in their weight groups, which determine how doctors treat patients. BMI, or the scale commonly used by medical practitioners, is a flawed method of determining health. BMI is not a perfect method of seeing how much body fat people have. Muscle weighs more than fat, so people who are muscular may be categorized as obese. A bodybuilder, for example, may weigh the same as someone who is obese but will have very little fat. Unfortunately, BMI continues to be used because doctors are still obsessed with the use of weight as a marker of health, which leads to the discrimination of heavier people in medical practices. To make matters worse, better methods have not been discovered for measuring fat, so while BMI often brings unnecessary shame onto people, it continues to be common in the medical community.

Myths being spread about larger bodies being bad are harmful to eating behaviors and how people function. When a whole society worships thin, even unhealthily thin bodies, it becomes easy to fantasize about whittling yourself down to a smaller size. People constantly stigmatize fat people, who are then made to feel like there's something wrong with them when the real sickness lies with society.

More than anything else, a culture of shaming people for their bodies can have adverse effects on the health and lifestyles of people. The societal pressures could be more harmful than extra weight. While higher BMIs have some association with reduced health, the actual health risks perpetrated may not be caused by the factors people commonly associate with obesity. Various researchers have argued that weight stigma, or the negative views and biases associated with weight, cause many of the health problems associated with being overweight. Common ideas that weight stigma perpetrates are that larger-bodied people are either lazy or simply don't have will power. This bias can be seen in individuals as young as three years old, showing how pervasive this phenomenon is our culture. In a well-known study from the 1950s, children were shown several images of other children and asked to rank them in order of which ones they liked best. The pictures included both "healthy" weight children and obese children. It also showed children with physical disabilities or facial disfigurements. In six groups of children who were of varying classes and races, the obese child came last in the ranking. In the time since that study, weight stigma has only become more deeply rooted in society.

Researchers suggest that it is this stigma that perpetuates the obesity "epidemic." Not only does this stigma make people spiral more out of control with their weight, but it makes them unable to be treated properly.

Additionally, weight stigma causes actual physiological changes in people. In studies, patients who were exposed to weight stigma ate more, were less able to self-regulate their eating, and had increases in cortisol levels (a hormone that is considered an obesogenic). People who experienced weight stigma were also less likely to engage in exercise, making weight maintenance even harder for them. They also have increased chances of mental health issues such as anxiety, being two times more likely to suffer anxiety and mood disorders.

The overall culture of dieting leads to binging, and it also creates great shame for those who binge. It took me years to choose recovery because I didn't realize how normal and societally induced my behaviors were. If there had been greater awareness around the topic and less stigma, I would have been able to share my problems with loved ones sooner and would have had support in getting better before my disorder got worse. You must share your struggles with at least one person in your life. Start breaking the stigma. By defying diet culture, you *can* have a happy and healthy life. It's important to understand, however, that you won't achieve it by counting calories.

Was I Born This Way?

Food and Your Childhood

You may wonder if you were born with your habits or if they were formed by how you grew up. Well, the answer is probably a little bit of both. Your DNA does factor into your binge eating, but your foundational experiences have a role of their own. Some people are predisposed to binge eating disorder based on genetics, but childhood trauma and strife can also be contributing factors. Studies have shown that negative childhood experiences have a considerable influence on eating patterns and obesity. Low-income childhoods as well, for example, can have a huge influence because those who have not had food security may be more likely to binge eat. Therefore, your childhood inevitably shapes your eating habits, so you must learn how your past influences your present. I hope you're ready for a deep dive into when you were a kid!

Examine how your parents treated food because many children learn their eating habits from their parents and carry on those habits into adulthood. Think about how your parents' food habits have been passed onto you or how you have resisted those habits they displayed. It should come as no surprise to you that you might be repeating those same patterns. Perhaps upon recollection, you realize that your dad was a binge eater, or you saw your mom overeating when she was anxious, so you started to eat when you were anxious, as well. These experiences cannot change the eating habits you've established, but they can highlight the areas that are most deeply rooted in your psyche.

Think about a moment when you felt free around food. Maybe you can't remember an *exact* time when you truly felt free with food, but many people can benefit from thinking back to a time when they ate what they wanted without feeling any shame or stigma. Remember how light and joyful you felt back then. Keep that feeling alive as you go through this journey because that's the feeling that you're looking to find yet again. Being mindful of your emotions is the key to progress.

Let go of the negative thoughts that you have internalized. Perhaps, from an early age, your grandma used to tell you that you needed to lose weight. Maybe you were bullied for your weight in school. Maybe you felt like you took up too much space because you were constantly degraded by someone you loved. Whatever negative thoughts that you're carrying, switch them out with positive ones because belittling yourself isn't going to help you stop binging.

Evaluate your eating history. Remember the times it made you feel good, and the times it made you feel bad. Think about when things went wrong with your eating. When did it change? Why did it change? Ask yourself about the emotional attachments that you have to food. In this process, you need to learn your triggers. Do you eat when you're bored? Angry? Anxious? Everyone has experiences that make them more prone to overeating, and many of these have roots in childhood. For example, your beloved aunt may have fed you cookies when you were feeling down, so now, in your adulthood, cookies still pacify you when you feel sad.

Let yourself move on from the past. Don't get stuck in the guilt and shame of things you couldn't control when you were a kid. Children often blame themselves for bad things that happen in their lives, and this blame can lead to continued self-blame if unaddressed. Be merciful with your childhood self. Back then, you were powerless, and you're not to blame for the bad done unto you by other people.

Work through your traumatic experiences. Stop ignoring your past if you haven't yet faced the things that hurt you when you were a child. If you have major traumatic experiences, consider therapy or, at least, find a friend who you feel safe talking to about hardships you've endured. If you still have old wounds, it's terribly hard to move forward, so make peace with what was so you can define what will be.

Know that you are more than your childhood experiences. You're much more than the person you used to be. You've learned, and you've grown. Focus on who you are now and the person you want to be in the future. Never forget the child who you were, but don't get stuck feeling small and helpless. You have the power now, and you can use that power to accomplish whatever you want to accomplish, including putting an end to binging for good.

Your Food Habits

Habits dictate much of what you do on any given day, but for the most part, they are unconscious, so it's easy to go about your day, not even being aware of the things you are doing simply because you're so used to doing them. Habits can be great to have because they allow you to accomplish tasks without having to exert as much mental energy, but when you have bad habits, it's hard to accomplish your goals, and it is easy to default to self-sabotage mode. Therefore, you need to curate food habits that help you move forward rather than walking in place.

Become aware of the habits that you have. The first step to any change is becoming aware of the processes that are normally unconscious to you. Make a list of habits that bother you. It helps to know all the things that trouble you the most. By writing a list of all your habits, you are becoming self-aware, which allows you to take the first step forward in shifting your life. Also, acknowledge the habits that you like. It's always good to look at what you're doing well because that helps keep you in a positive headspace.

Don't let your habits define you. Just because you eat a lot of sugar, doesn't in any way make you a bad person. Your food habits have nothing to do with your character. Moreso, they are related to your DNA and your tastes. Wanting to change something doesn't mean that thing is bad as it is. Wanting to wear a different outfit doesn't mean you hated the last one you had on, and the same can be said concerning healthy eating habits. Instilling more nutrient-dense food in your diet doesn't mean that your old diet habits were bad; it just means that you're making a change that reflects the dynamic needs of your body and mind.

Understand that habits can be changed. Don't let yourself feel defeated just because you have some bad habits. I'll talk more about how to instill good habits later, but the short of it is that habits can be changed. It takes time to change them, which causes many people to give up on changing prior habits when they've only just started making progress. Nevertheless, an old dog can always be taught new tricks, do dedicate yourself to making change because that's the best way to ensure that change will *actually happen*. It also helps that I'm not asking you to make drastic changes. Every habit you swap out will feel relatively easy. Just like you aren't defined solely by your childhood experiences, you don't have to be defined by your habits either, so accept your old habits while embracing your new ones too.

Food and Your Emotions

The hardest part to deal with when it comes to binge eating is your emotional connection to food. You're never going to stop having one, and that's okay, because you don't have to steer clear of the foods that make you feel good. You'll always have memories related to food, and trying to change those memories would be a waste of time.

Even now, after being free from food worries for so many years, I still have an emotional connection to food. I don't let that connection drive my life, but some things cannot and should not be severed. For instance, I still have fond memories associated with my mom's gingerbread dough that we'd roll out and cut into shapes to make dozens of fun cookies. Similarly, chocolate cake with mint icing will always remind me of my dad. I can't help but grin a little when I eat it, although, I would never binge either of those foods anymore. I no longer feel the need to because I've learned to respect the emotional connection I have to food, which allows me to eat in moderation.

It may take you a while to get to where I am. It took me months to get rid of binge eating together, but there are ways you can become more cognizant of your emotional connection to food. Make a list of foods that give you comfort, and these foods should be the first that you stop restricting. Eat them even if it feels scary to do so. Give your body what it wants so that it can get better.

Know that it's okay to use food as a source of joy. Eat things that you love! Make your favorite recipes and share your food traditions with your kids. Having peace with food means that you can love it again. It doesn't have to be something you both love and hate all at once. You can even find new ways to love food. Try foods you've never let yourself taste before. Experiment with new cuisines and take the limits off yourself. You don't need to be uncomfortable around food any longer.

Social experiences shouldn't make you feel nervous just because food is there. Social encounters can be hard when you binge eat because just being around food can make you feel like you're going to lose control. You don't realize how many social events are centered around food until food starts to become the enemy. When I was in college, there were countless times when I blew off my friends just because they were going somewhere that had a lot of food. I couldn't go to a buffet without feeling like I was going to completely lose control over the situation. I stopped enjoying my experiences with the people I loved, and when I did go out with them, my time was ruined by all the worrying I did over food. I felt so disconnected from everyone because I was trapped in my head. It was remarkable how much more engaged I became when I stopped binge eating. It was as if a switch had flipped, and I was finally free to be me again. I could enjoy being social without that constant worry that binge eating might be linked to it. I want you to find the same liberation and be able to go out and have fun.

Trust in your body to make sure you don't go too overboard when you indulge rather than trying to control your eating with restriction. I will warn you that it will take your body some time to realize that you are not going to deprive it. You may have the urge to binge for months after you've started making changes, but that's okay. This is a process, so it's not going to shift overnight. Don't get discouraged if you even gain weight when you first start eating more mindfully because your weight will fluctuate a bit before reaching into its set point.

Food and your emotions will never be fully disconnected, so relinquish the control you're trying to have over your hunger and let yourself experience food without limiting how much you can enjoy it. Nothing should be off-limits anymore because limits only lead to binges.

Chapter 2:
Slow Down and Silence The Urge

Eat Slowly and on Purpose

Mealtimes shouldn't be something that you rush through just to get them done. Take your time with meals so that your body can digest food properly as you learn to feel satiated and eat your meals with purpose. Always know why you are eating and give your full attention to the mealtime so that you can upkeep positive habits and look upon meals with positivity and joy. You need to learn to love food again and enjoy every bite you take. If you're not, there's a good chance you are not eating with respect to your body.

Why Eating Slowly Helps

Diet books have long advocated for eating slowly, and there's science backing up how beneficial it can be. While this book has an incredibly different goal than weight loss books, I agree that there are several benefits to eating at a moderate pace. In short, eating slowly can make you feel full faster, and it also helps you break from the typical binge behavior of eating too quickly, which allows you to be more mindful when you are eating.

Eating slowly gives your hunger signals time to kick in. It takes around twenty minutes before your body can recognize that it is full, so by eating slowly, you can better read your hunger signals and be in tune with how much food you need. When you eat too quickly, your body just isn't ready to keep up with you because the necessary processes and release of chemicals takes time.

You digest your food more easily when you eat slowly. Your GI tract works using a step by step process. At the beginning of this process, you begin to salivate when you smell the food or even just think about it. From there, you begin to eat the food, and it starts to break down in your mouth using saliva as well as chewing. As you start eating, your stomach needs to prepare for the food that is coming and prepare digestive acids. Accordingly, if you eat too quickly, you're forcing your digestive system to operate before it is adequately prepared, which is why eating slowly can give your system a better chance at properly digesting your food.

People who eat more slowly feel more content post meals. In a study by the University of Rhode Island, researchers found that women who ate meals faster not only ate more calories, but they felt less lasting satisfaction after eating. So, by eating slowly, you will be able to appreciate your food and feel more satiated until your next meal.

Research suggests that the pace in which you eat matters, so don't shovel all your food into your mouth as quickly as possible when you are eating. Mealtimes don't need to be rushed, so let yourself savor the meal that's in front of you so that you don't wind up binging later when you feel unsatisfied because you didn't get the enjoyment you wanted from your food.

Enjoy Your Meal

If you're not enjoying your food, you're never going to feel satisfied because you are not fulfilling your needs. When I was binging, I never enjoyed my food. I loved the taste of it, but in a binge, I barely tasted anything. The food glided over my taste buds, slithering down my throat before I could even appreciate it. When you're eating at lightning speed and simply trying to get as much food into yourself as possible, you're not focusing on the tastes and textures of what you're eating. You're wasting the experience of eating by not truly enjoying it.

Don't eat foods that you hate no matter how nutritious they are. If you don't like certain vegetables or fruits, don't eat them! Eating foods that you don't like will only make you crave foods that you do like more and lead to binging. Find alternatives for the foods that you don't like so that it never feels like you're forcing yourself to eat anything that you absolutely despise.

Allow yourself treats. When you crave something, eat it. Don't eat it and then punish yourself later by restricting what you have at your next meal. Just eat and don't make a big deal out of the calories or nutritional facts. There's nothing wrong with having the foods that most delight you when the urge strikes. When you let yourself eat these foods, you won't want to binge them because you won't feel deprived. Enjoyment is key in healing from binge eating, so cutting out your favorite treats is counterproductive.

Try new recipes, and don't let your meals become too stagnant. When you eat the same thing every day, meals can get incredibly boring. Thus, you need to try different foods whenever you can. You need to make sure that mealtimes are something you enjoy having. I'm sure that you have enough stress during your day, so you need time when you can relax and enjoy your food. Make it a priority to sit down for meals and savor the food you are eating because it will make a dramatic difference in your progress.

How to Eat With Purpose

Eating should never be something that you do just because. Eat with intention. For each meal you have, you should remain in the moment and mindful of the meal that is in front of you. When you binge eat, it's easy to lose purpose when it comes to meals. You become so used to eating massive quantities that eating stops being special and even feels like a chore at times. Find your purpose in meals to reinvigorate your joy of eating.

Don't eat while distracted. Eating shouldn't be done in front of your TV, and you shouldn't be trying to eat while you work. Eating should be an activity all of its own. It's okay to eat with other people and talk during your meal because that's part of the mealtime experience, but doing activities that distract you from the purpose of your meal isn't helpful.

Make time for meals. We all have busy lives, but you need to prioritize meals. They're incredibly important because meals keep you alive. Don't let yourself skip meals just because you get busy. That's not a good enough excuse. Eat meals and have snacks when you feel hungry between meals. If you want to get better, you have to dedicate the appropriate time to your meals because making sure your hunger is respected as one of the best things you can do for yourself. Respect your hunger by letting it be fed promptly.

Don't be afraid to make meals a social experience. Get your loved ones involved in making mealtimes feel more focused. Eating alone can be triggering and feel like it's not worth the time, so whenever you can, try to bring people you enjoy being around into the experience of eating. Sharing meals is one of the most rewarding activities that humans can do. Breaking bread with others has deep cultural significance, so a meal often feels more like a meal when other people are around. Having other people around helps structure a meal, giving it a beginning and an end, but also, the company of other people can be a great distraction from any troubling food thoughts.

Never count calories. Ever. If you have an app on your phone, delete it right now. There's no reason to keep track of what you are eating that specifically. Not only are people inaccurate when they calorie count, but calorie counting apps will never know the needs of your body, as well as your body does. Don't stress yourself out with numbers that don't even matter. Let yourself be calm and free from worrying about how much you are eating.

Be grateful for what your meal has provided for you. Whatever in life guides you, be thankful for your nourishment and the meal you have. Gratitude is a great tool and allows people to feel more optimistic and have a positive outlook on life.

Remind yourself of all the good things that the food is doing for your body. Food allows you to talk to your friends, work, read, laugh, and a million other activities. Everything you do requires energy, so eat with that purpose in mind. Envision all the things that food will allow you to do. Eating with purpose takes time to master, but it's well worth the effort.

The Benefits of Keeping a Food Journal

Too many people dismiss the usefulness of a journal, but journaling is one of the most helpful daily activities that you can do for a myriad of reasons. Those who journal are better able to make changes in their lives. Not only do people who journal feel better about their situation, they also are overall healthier people. Maybe you doubt how effective journaling is, but let me highlight some of the key benefits, and I'll see if I can change your mind.

Keep in mind that your food journal should be much more than just what you're eating. I also want you to note how you are feeling. Feel free to include things that seem unrelated to food— like an issue you have at work— because even the smallest things can influence your food behavior and lead up to a binge. With that in mind, write as much as your day in your journal as you'd like. The more information, the better.

Journaling has been shown to have several health benefits, and I'm not just talking about mental health benefits. Not only is it a great stress reliever, but journaling for just fifteen minutes three days a week has been shown to lower people's blood pressure. Journaling is also beneficial to your memory. It helps you comprehend the world around you better and also improve your cognitive processing. If that's not enough, those who journal, get sick less often because studies have shown that people who can express themselves through words can improve their immune system. The simple act of journaling can improve conditions such as asthma or arthritis, showing how miraculous utilizing your brain in the right ways can be.

People who journal are also happier. Those who are in the habit of journaling benefit from being able to handle their moods better. People who can be self-reflective can better engage in the world and be more creative in their everyday lives. Thus, journaling leads to people feeling more confident in their skills and creative abilities.

When you keep a journal, you're holding yourself accountable. You're not allowing yourself to put off recovery until tomorrow. You're forcing yourself to live up to what you accomplish. You need that accountability to ensure that you stay in line and don't start fooling yourself. I used to fool myself a lot. I'd convince myself that I could start getting better tomorrow, but then tomorrow came, and I would binge again and vow that tomorrow would be different. It never was until I finally decided that I needed to take charge of my life and stop letting myself get away with hurting myself. I had a moment of realizing that I had to start holding myself responsible for my actions, or I'd be living in binging and dieting torment forever.

Research shows that people who write stuff down are more likely to accomplish goals and complete what they have written down, showing how journaling can influence your mindset. A survey taken by Harvard Business Study shows that eighty-three percent of people have no goals while fourteen percent of people had goals that they didn't write down. Only a mere three percent of people wrote down their goals. Correspondingly, in a study by the Dominican University of California, that groups who wrote down their goals had increased odds of achieving them.

Writing down things such as your food intake and how you feel when you eat can help you identify patterns in your behavior. When you write stuff down, you become conscious of it. Many of our food behaviors are unconscious. We do them out of habit, meaning that we easily lose sight of what we're doing to ourselves. The longer you keep your journal, the more you will learn about yourself. I've had countless moments of realization when writing in my journal. It's almost as good as therapy!

By keeping a journal, you can feel in control of your life without having to manipulate your eating. A journal can be a place to vent all the things that make you feel out of control. You can take the power back by working through your problems instead of continuing to avoid them. Avoidance isn't a tactic you can afford to use anymore. It's time to face up to your feelings and behaviors.

Don't be obsessive about counting calories. The goal of journaling is not to fixate on quantity. I want you to keep your food talk in your journal vague. It's good to write down what you're eating, but instead of quantifying what you are eating, I want you to try qualifying it. Instead of writing, for example, "25 chips- 150 calories," I want you to describe those chips, "delicious kettle-cooked barbeque chips that satisfied my craving." Be honest with what foods you are eating, but be sure to include how you are feeling as well. If you feel unsatisfied with a certain food you've eaten, don't be afraid to admit that. When you binge, write that down. There's no point in lying to your journal or yourself. You're the only one in the world who is going to read it, so don't be ashamed about being honest.

Journaling can be beneficial for anyone, but it is especially beneficial for people who desperately need to promote change in their lives. It takes less than half an hour a day to make meaningful changes in your life through your journal. Even if you're still skeptical, it's worth a shot. It can't hurt, can it?

Instant Gratification Is the Enemy

What Is Instant Gratification?

Instant gratification is receiving an immediate reward for your actions. Many people expect instant results. They want their reward right away rather than waiting for it to come in the future. Instant gratification is one of the reasons why binging feels so good. When you binge, the second that food hits your mouth, you get the great sensation of tasting food that was once off-limits. You don't wait to be gratified, and as you eat, you keep wanting more of that gratification. However, nothing feels as good as that first bite. You become addicted to that first wonderful sensation and keep chasing it as you binge and binge.

The neuroscience behind instant gratification makes sense. Instant gratification gives our brains a different feeling than a delayed reward does, and the delayed reward often doesn't give us the same rush of overwhelming happiness that instant results do. The brain understands immediacy well. If you fall on your arm and your arm is broken, you know why your arm is broken. The pain you are experiencing makes perfect sense, but if you didn't feel that pain until a month later, you'd be a lot more confused about why your arm is hurting. Therefore, it makes sense for us to experience things right away, and it's harder to think in the long-term.

One quintessential experiment nicely shows the role of instant gratification in decision-making. The Stanford Marshmallow Experiment is one of the most well-known experiments of all time. In this experiment, young children around five-years of age were sat in rooms with marshmallows on the table in front of them. The children were told that they could eat their marshmallows right away, but if the children waited until the researcher left and came back into the room that they could have second marshmallows. After leaving the room for fifteen minutes, the researcher came back, and some kids ate the marshmallows as soon as the researcher left the room while others waited a little longer. A few were able to wait the full time. The experiment then followed the children for forty years to find patterns among those who were able to delay gratification and those who weren't.

The children who were able to delay their gratification grew up to have better test scores, were less likely to abuse substances, had better social skills, were less obese, and could better manage stress. Interestingly, these children had been divided into groups, and one group was promised crayons and then never got them while the second group was given the crayons that they were told they would get. The children who had learned that they couldn't trust that they would get what they were promised, tended to eat the marshmallows more often.

The same concepts come into play in binge eating. When you restrict your food intake, your body believes that it is not going to receive the food that it expects, so you binge, and your body is resistant to receiving any delayed reaction. Many people who experience binge eating disorder may have a harder time with impulse control, meaning that instant gratification can seem even more appealing. Research has suggested that overeating is often caused by a lack of long-term thinking, which makes it hard for people to resist the marvelous tastes of food that they could have right now.

Why Is Instant Gratification Bad?

The need for instant gratification can be counterproductive to your progress because it allows your potentially destructive impulses to take control of your actions rather than letting you make clear, controlled decisions. You stop being in control and the instant gratification becomes the decision-maker. Don't let instant gratification be the thing that defines how you behave. You don't need to give in to your impulses. Instead, with a little practice, you can let yourself be future thinking.

Unfortunately, instant gratification causes you to act before you think. You find yourself diving headfirst into a bag of chips before you can think any better of it. I've been there hundreds of times. When I binged, it would feel as though I was in a trance, and I no longer felt like I was making my own decisions. I'd start eating, promising that I'd have just one taste, but then, knowing that I was just going to restrict my food intake again, I kept eating. I figured that I was already ruining my diet, so I might as well make the most of it. I gave into my immediate urges and rationalized them instead of considering what doing so might do to future me.

Instant gratification also prolongs how long you have to wait to get results. Instant gratification makes you put off lasting change by tearing your focus from your goals. You constantly focus on what you can do to feel good now rather than what you can do to feel good permanently. Instant gratification makes you put things off until tomorrow because you're too focused on what you can receive today.

Instant gratification doesn't give you long-term satisfaction. Binging doesn't feel good. It makes your body ache, your throat hurt, and your lips dry from all the salt and sugar you've eaten. It makes you feel a bit hungover— a headache and nausea overcomes you as the food finally settles. Mentally, you don't feel any better. You feel ashamed and angry at yourself for messing up yet again. You get caught up in a self-pitying spiral, and no matter what you do, you feel disgusted at your behaviors. Binging often feels good as you're doing it, but then the appeal wears off, and you feel worse than you did before.

You'll never accomplish anything in the future if you're only looking at what you can get out of today. You need to stop seeking instant gratification because it will never give you the long-term satisfaction that I'm sure you want. It will be hard, but you can use a few simple tips to help yourself look ahead instead of getting caught up in the moment.

How to Avoid Striving for Instant Gratification

Don't expect results right away. You're not going to stop binging overnight. Your body needs time to adjust to the changes you are making and realize that you are not continuing your unhealthy relationship with food. Once your body feels secure and knows that you are going to take care of it, it will start to fall into place, and you'll have the urge to binge at lessening frequency. In time, you will be free of binging altogether, and your set point weight will be restored.

Visualize the future. Visualization is a great tool to make what you want to happen in the future come true. Psychologists have found that visualization is an impactful technique that anyone can do from the comfort of their own home. High performing athletes, celebrities and billionaires have all used visualization to make their dreams come true. Imagine yourself in the future, holding your favorite food. Now imagine a monster looming behind you, pestering you to eat that food. Visualize yourself, checking in with your hunger, and realizing that you aren't hungry. Finally, visualize yourself telling the binge monster that you don't want your favorite food and hand over the food to him. By imagining what can happen in the future, you're setting yourself up for success and giving yourself a taste of what you can look forward to.

Remind yourself what you're fighting for. Never forget why you want to quit binging. Remember all the agony and discomfort that your binge eating has put you through. Think of your lowest moments and keep remembering not just how far you have to go but how far you have come in your binge eating journey. By remembering what you don't want to go back to, you will have the motivation to carry on, even if the results aren't instantaneous.

Make daily goals. Incremental goals will help you find gratification each day. As you wake up every day, make a to-do list of the things that you would like to accomplish. Keep it simple so that you don't overwhelm yourself, but make sure that you have tasks to check off your to-do list. Completing these small tasks will make your long-term goals feel more manageable. One thing you can do is say, 'I will not binge today," and that seems a lot more manageable than saying, "I will never binge again," right at the start of your journey. Most people can't just stop on day one. If they could, they would have done it by now, so don't expect to *never* binge again. Slip-ups happen, and it's okay.

Find victory in little things. Any progress you make shouldn't be scoffed at or minimized. Not binging for one day when you usually binge every day is an amazing step forward. It may not seem like much, but that's more than what many people do. Know that waiting for the reward will get you the best results and embrace the waiting. Let the journey give you joy rather than just the destination.

Listen to Your Body

The human body is an incredible thing, and your body will give you vital information that keeps your hunger at a manageable level and allows you to eat food without fear, but you have to learn to accept and translate that information based on what your body is saying. You need to be able to evaluate both your health and your hunger if you want to ensure that you are staying on the right track.

Evaluating Your Health

Be aware of the changes happening in your body. Note what makes you feel better and what makes you feel worse so that you can more easily make changes that you can stick to. Keeping healthy is a dynamic experience, meaning that you have to check in with yourself. When your body starts to feel a little bit out of synch, adjust and see what tweaks you can make to make it feel better. Some days your body may be more exhausted than others, for example, and when you are tired, you may be more prone to overeating. Thus, listening to the cues that your body gives you, like yawning and aching, can help you counteract your hunger.

Know your body's limits. Maybe you have a physical ailment or intolerances of certain foods. Keep these ideas in mind so that you don't do anything that makes it harder to stick to good habits. Take care of yourself when you don't feel well. If you have not been running, don't get up and try to run a marathon. Exercise can be a great tool for channeling excess energy, but if you're taking on too much at once, you're only going to get yourself hurt. Be gentle with yourself.

Make sure your nutrition matches your health needs. Certain foods can benefit people with select conditions. If you have any chronic conditions, do some research on foods that can help alleviate some of your pain or other symptoms. Don't restrict anything that your body needs to function. If you're having cravings, they may be a sign of what your body needs. Your body often craves foods that contain essential nutrients, so listen to your cravings when they arise.

Remember that without your health, you can never have happiness. While the way your body looks doesn't matter, how it functions is vital. Your brain can't accomplish what it wants if your body isn't up for it. Your body should be something you value, and when you value your body, you treat it well. You don't put it through unnecessary hardships or ignore its signals. Learn to respect your body and its abilities regardless of what size that body is. As soon as you can do that, you'll be able to accomplish true inner peace.

Evaluating Your Hunger

If you can evaluate your hunger, you will be able to maintain healthy eating patterns without having to use rigid diets that only make you feel worse about yourself and your condition. Understanding your hunger will give you the tools you need to understand what your body requires to function optimally. Learn to observe your hunger cues and to become fully aware of not only that your body needs food, but what *kind* of food it needs. Of course, doing that can seem overwhelming, and it takes extensive practice, but there are several ways in which you can gauge your hunger and get more in touch with your body.

Strive for intuitive eating, but don't let yourself get overwhelmed by expecting to be able to eat intuitively right away. It takes time to transition. Intuitive eating is a concept with several principles that help people get in touch with their hunger signals. Intuitive eating includes people of all sizes and resists diet culture. Intuitive eating allows you to eat whatever you want as long as you are listening to what your body is saying. It teaches you not to see food as good or bad, but to see the gradient nature of food and that any food is okay to eat so long as you recognize when you are full.

Learn to rank your hunger until you can eat intuitively without thought. The use of a hunger scale can help you determine whether your desire to eat is rooted in actual hunger or is a physical need. Commonly, hunger scales rank hunger from a level of one, which is ravenous for food, to ten, which indicates that you feel so sick you can't eat anything more. Meanwhile, a seven would represent when you feel totally satisfied and a level four is when your hunger first begins. The other numbers fall somewhere between. Make a scale with rankings that fit you. You can define what levels of hunger stand out most to you. You can use your scale before and after meals to check in with yourself on what your body needs. Using a scale will help you identify emotional hunger from physical hunger.

The hunger scale method is straightforward, but it can be hard at first because you may be out of touch with your body. But the more you use it, the more natural it will become until you can intuitively know when you need food and when you should stop eating.

An example of a hunger scale is as follows:

1. You're feeling dizzy, shaky, or weak.
2. You're struggling to pay attention and are moody.
3. You're starting to feel uncomfortable because of your hunger.
4. You're beginning to feel hungry.
5. You're currently content, but you could have more food.
6. You're not hungry or full.
7. You're satisfied but starting to get full.
8. You're starting to feel bloated and overly full.

9. Your clothes are starting to feel constrictive.
10. You're so full that you feel sick.

Respect your hunger. Your hunger is something that you cannot change. It exists within you, and not letting that hunger exist means ignoring all the problems associated with that hunger, as well as, all the joys.

Chapter 3:

Improve Your Nutrition, Improve Your Life

What Are My Daily Nutritional Requirements?

There are certain foods you should make sure that you have daily. The World Health Organization has suggested that twenty nutrients are deemed necessary for health, which includes micronutrients, fat-soluble vitamins, thiamine, niacin, riboflavin, vitamin B6, pantothenic acid, iodine, magnesium, zinc, biotin, vitamin B12, vitamin C, calcium, antioxidants, and folate. These are all important for optimal human function, among others.

The nutrients that you put in your body are vital to your health, and if you are not healthy, you will not be able to stop binging. Therefore, learn what foods you should be eating to get all the nutrients you need and learn the pains and problems that may occur when you don't.

The United States Department of Agriculture suggests that people try to find foods that are a modest portion, are nutritionally dense, and are varied. Furthermore, it emphasizes making small, incremental changes to improve your health. Nevertheless, the USDA, just like me, says that our specific circumstances influence what we eat and that each person will have plates that look unique. There are, however, certain foods that nutritionists would urge you to be sure to include in your diet. The first category you need to learn about are macronutrients, which make up the caloric content of your food and give you energy. Macronutrients include carbs, proteins, and fats. Alcohol is a less nutritionally necessary macronutrient that contains seven calories per gram.

Carbs

Carbs are maybe one of the most controversial macronutrients. You can probably identity some foods that contain carbs such as cookies, cake, and bread, but you may be less clear on what a carb is. Carbohydrates, commonly referred to as just carbs, are created using carbon, hydrogen, and oxygen. Carbs have four calories per gram. On average, people need about 135 grams of carbs per day, but each person will have distinctive needs based on their weight and how much energy they use. For example, a diabetic may want to limit carbs to ensure they remain under a certain number while a pregnant woman may require more carbs than average. Generally, you should aim to have forty-five to sixty-five percent of your caloric content be made up of carbs.

You need to have carbs daily unless you are told to cut back for medical reasons (a keto diet, which is a low carb diet, can be used to help people with epilepsy and other disorders in select cases). Your body uses carbs to provide energy to working muscles, as well as your central nervous system. They also make sure your muscles aren't used to fuel your body and allow your fat to metabolize. Carbs are also the preferred energy source of your brain. In the absence of carbs, the body can convert fat into ketones in a process called ketosis, but the body is built to fuel your brain using carbs, making them essential to your body.

Carbs often have a bad reputation in the world of dieting. They are often treated as unhealthy and fattening when that couldn't be further from the truth. What people do not realize is that not all carbs are created equally. There are two categories of carbs: simple carbs and complex carbs. Simple carbs are the carbs that are often vilified by diets. While you shouldn't eliminate them completely from your diet, you should know that these carbs do not make you feel as satiated because they are digested more quickly. Further, simple carbs will lead to your energy levels crashing quickly. They also tend to have reduced nutrition because fiber-filled portions have been removed. Complex carbs, meanwhile, are polysaccharides meaning that they have at least three sugars in them, whereas simple carbs only have two. Complex carbs make you feel energized longer and satiated. Foods such as whole grains, potatoes, and legumes are examples of complex carbs. It is important to add more complex carbs to your diet for better health outcomes. Research has suggested that eating carbs instead of saturated fats can reduce your risk of heart disease and diabetes.

People who do not have enough carbs in their diet will likely feel changes in their bodies. You may start to feel moodier and have trouble concentrating or remembering. When you don't have enough carbs, your decision-making skills may also suffer, making it harder to maintain good dietary decisions as the day drags on. Thus, try to include complex carbs in your diet so that you can feel happy and healthy.

Proteins

Proteins are the macronutrient that people tend to rank with the most fondness, and for good reason. They have four calories per gram. While all macronutrients are important in a balanced diet, proteins are a jack-of-all-trades and help your body carry out an expanse of functions. The jobs of fats and carbs are more focused, while proteins have roles in several processes. Protein is made of nitrogen, which makes the amino acids that form proteins. Some amino acids can be made within your body, while others must be obtained from food sources. The former group is called non-essential amino acids, while the latter are essential amino acids. There are nine essential amino acids that you need to be healthy. All animal-based proteins will contain all nine of these. Eleven amino acids can be produced by your body if you are getting other nutrients that you need.

Dieters and those who want to gain muscle often love protein because protein can be great in helping you gain muscle, but it also has a myriad of other functions. Protein helps your body break down the food you're eating, repair tissues throughout your body, and make enzymes. It is also one of the main building blocks for things such as your bones, skin, blood, hair, and cartilage.

Focus on lean proteins. Chicken, turkey, 90% lean ground beef, beans, lentils, low fat or skim dairy, salmon, tuna, tuna, and egg whites are all examples of lean proteins, which are proteins that have less than ten grams of fat per serving. Proteins can be found in animal products like dairy, eggs, and meat. They also can be found in plant-based products. Foods like quinoa, amaranth, and buckwheat are nearly complete protein sources. Though, the only complete protein source that is plant-based is soybeans, which are found in products like tofu; however, you can use complementary proteins to make up a full protein that has all the amino acids that you need. Certain proteins can be paired together to add up to a full source. There are three groups of plant-based proteins, and from these groups, you must choose two foods from two distinct categories to get a complete protein. You may choose from grains, legumes, or nuts and seeds. Thus, eating black beans with whole grain rice would provide you a full protein serving. Alternatively, oatmeal and peanut butter would also give you a complete serving.

Eat proteins throughout the day. Whereas your body can store fats and carbs to varying degrees, your body does not store proteins. Thus, it helps to eat several meals and snacks throughout the day, each with protein sources. You shouldn't strive to eat as much protein as possible because your body can only use so much. Generally, men should try to have three servings of protein, totaling to six to seven ounces while women, children, and teenagers can aim to have as little as two servings that contain five to six ounces of protein. The amount you need will depend on your activity level. Burn victims, for example, need additional protein because their bodies have extensive reparations to do.

Being deficient in protein can cause several unhealthy effects on your body. When you lack the proper protein, you may suffer from protein-energy malnutrition (PEM). PEM, in severe cases called kwashiorkor, happens when people do not get enough protein in their diet. These people may be getting the proper caloric value that they need but do not have the protein levels needed for their body to function or even process the food that they are eating. It is commonly seen in countries that are experiencing famine, making it hard for people to get balanced diets. It is also common in alcoholics, who get many calories from alcohol and therefore do not have enough protein. Malnourished people, for example, sometimes experience extra swelling in their bodies— in their feet, stomachs, and ankles— because of the dysfunction caused by a lack of protein. Thus, protein is crucial to your health and ability to be healthy.

Fats

Fats are one of the foods that worry people the most. At nine calories per gram, they are the most calorically dense food, which makes people fear that eating fats will lead to weight gain. Like carbs, fats are frequently misunderstood. The bottom line, though, is that your body needs fat to function. Of course, having too much isn't helpful, but without fat, your body won't be able to keep your organs protected. Fat is responsible for giving your body back up energy that it can burn when the energy provided by carbs has run out. When you exercise, you will start burning fat about twenty minutes into your workout.

Your body needs fats for more than just having energy at the ready for when you're running low on carbs. It's also crucial that you have dietary fat so fat-soluble vitamins like K, D, A and E be absorbed. These vitamins help your hair and skin stay healthy, maintain your vision and support your immune system. They also ensure that your reproductive system works, bones are healthy, and help your blood clot properly. In addition to allowing you to absorb vitamins, fat insulates your body and protects your organs. When your body doesn't have enough fat to fuel you, it will start to break down muscle for energy, including heart muscles, which can lead to issues such as heart failure. Disallowing any fat from your diet is ultimately dangerous to your wellbeing. Aim to ensure fat makes up anywhere from twenty to thirty-five percent of your caloric intake and saturated fat makes up under ten percent of your daily calories.

Some fats are better for you than others. Listed in order from least to most healthy, there are three kinds of fats: trans fats, saturated fats, monounsaturated fats and polyunsaturated fats. It is important to focus on incorporating more healthy fats and less of the others.

Generally, you want to avoid trans fats whenever possible. Trans fats do extensive damage to your health. They increase levels of LDL cholesterol in your blood (which is the bad cholesterol) and decrease how much HDL cholesterol is in your blood (which is the cholesterol that is good for you). Trans fats can also cause inflammation, lead to insulin resistance, cause heart problems, and worsen chronic conditions. One startling statistic from Harvard Health suggests that eating just two percent of calories in trans fat correlates to an increased risk of heart disease. While many countries, including the United States, have banned trans fats, companies can still put trans fat into their foods as long as they are less than 0.5 grams per serving. Fortunately, the number of products with trans fats is decreasing. Some foods like dairy and meat may have limited naturally occurring trans fats, which studies have shown to be less harmful than synthetic trans fats (commonly found in microwavable popcorn, vegetable shortening, fast food, and snack cakes).

Saturated fats aren't as toxic as trans fats, but they should be eaten in moderation. They increase LDL cholesterol, which can cause blockages in your body, so too many can be incredibly harmful. They are found in foods like red meat, full-fat dairy, and many highly processed foods. Don't deprive yourself of these foods but swap out this kind of fat as much as you can for a better health outcome. The better your body feels, the easier it will be not to binge.

Monounsaturated fats and polyunsaturated fats are both excellent for your health. To show how good these fats are, research from the 1960s has shown that despite having a lot of fat in their diets, Greek people who followed the Mediterranean diet had decreased risks of heart disease even though fat was an important part of their eating style. The key was that they ate a plethora of monounsaturated fats such as olive oil, avocados, nuts, safflower oil, and sunflower oil.

Polyunsaturated fats are another type of fat that you need to include in your diet because they are essential fats. These fats not only reduce bad cholesterol, but they can increase good cholesterol. They also reduce the number of triglycerides in your blood. Triglycerides are formed when you eat more calories than you need to use. These lipids being in your blood can lead to heart problems and other health conditions when you have too many. There are two predominant types: omega-three fatty acids and omega-six fatty acids. Omega-threes increase good cholesterol and can help your heart rhythm and reduce your chance for stroke. They could also help with conditions such as arthritis. These fatty acids can be found in cold-water fish like tuna and salmon. They are also found in flaxseeds, canola oil, soybean oil, and certain nuts like walnuts. Omega-six fatty acids are also good for your heart, and they can be found in various vegetable oils like safflower, sunflower, or corn oils.

When your body is deficient in fats, you are unable to have the proper energy stores you need to function and unable to appropriately absorb important fat-soluble vitamins. Therefore, you should try to include healthy fats as often as you can in your diet as opposed to less healthy ones.

Micronutrients

While carbs, proteins, and fats are macronutrients, you should be eating every day; micronutrients include vitamins and minerals that you need to be including in your diet to make sure that you are functioning optimally. Compared to macronutrients, you don't need as high quantities of these in your body, but that doesn't make them any less important. Micronutrients are often found in fruits and vegetables. Naturally colorful foods tend to be packed with nutritional value, and the colors of the foods often correlate to what kind of vitamins they contain, so make sure you're eating a variety of foods.

Some people may need more micronutrients than others. Pregnant women, for instance, need many vitamins to stay healthy. Getting vitamins through food is preferable, but supplements can help those who cannot acquire all their vitamins through their meals.

Fat-Soluble Vitamins

These vitamins, as I've already mentioned, need fat to be absorbed. When consumed, they are stored in your body so that you can use them later. Here is a breakdown of these vitamins and how they affect your body.

Vitamin K is found in leafy greens like spinach and kale, broccoli, milk, cabbage, eggs, soybeans, and pumpkin. It helps your blood clot and helps your bones. Without vitamin K, you may have hemorrhaging, and the calcium in your bones may lessen.

Vitamin E is predominantly found in leafy greens, whole grains, almonds (and other nuts), and vegetable oils. It acts like an antioxidant, is good for your cells, and helps with your immune system. If you're deficient in vitamin E, you may experience anemia, weakened muscles, and hemorrhaging.

Vitamin D helps you absorb calcium so that your bones are healthy. It also improves your immune function. Vitamin D is unique in that you can get it from the sun, but using sun protection (which you should be using) will block the rays needed for vitamin D absorption, and colder climates might not get the necessary sunlight for this vitamin.

Luckily, it can be found in other foods like fortified milk and cereals. It's also in some fish like salmon and mackerel. Without vitamin D, you may have soft bones and osteomalacia.

Vitamin A is good for your vision and your organs. Deficiency, however, can lead to vision problems, including blindness or night blindness. This vitamin is found in seafood like shrimp, fortified milk, carrots, mangoes, spinach, beef, eggs, and sweet potatoes.

Water-Saluble Vitamins

These vitamins are not stored by the body, so you need to eat them regularly in your diet. There are eight B vitamins and one C vitamin in this group.

Thiamin (B1) is commonly found in pork, fish, and poultry. It is also found in whole grains, nuts, legumes as well as enriched cereals. Thiamin aids in regulating the body's appetite. It also aids in the process of turning carbohydrates into energy. When you don't have enough of thiamin, you may get a condition called beriberi. As a result, you could have muscle weakness, edema, heart irregularities, and mental fogginess.

Riboflavin (B2) is a vitamin that also helps process carbohydrates as well as fats and proteins. It also ensures that your skin is healthy, and your vision is clear. It is found in dairies like milk, cottage cheese, and yogurt. It is also found in leafy green vegetables, meats, and enriched foods. Without this micronutrient, you may experience eye issues, tongue discoloration, and light hypersensitivity. One tell-tale sign of a riboflavin deficiency is skin problems in the nose and mouth areas.

Niacin (B3) is yet another one that helps with the release of energy. It also helps keep your skin clear, as well as, keeping your nerves and digestive system functioning at their best. Even more importantly, it allows you to create your sex hormones and stress-relieving hormones. You can get this vitamin through most protein sources like meat, fish, eggs, whole grains, enriched cereals, and peanuts. While niacin is not in all these foods directly, your body can convert the amino acid, tryptophan, into niacin. Without it, you may experience a condition called pellagra and have a loss of appetite. You may also experience delirium, flaky skin, be moody, and have indigestion. Most people in the developed world do not experience this deficiency. However, alcoholics may experience it more often.

Pantothenic Acid (B5) can be found in a wide range of foods such as broccoli, mushrooms, chicken, or whole grains, and you need it for fatty acid synthesis to occur. People usually don't become deficient in this nutrient, but in cases when people don't get enough, they might have trouble sleeping, feel sick, and be tired.

Pyridoxine (B6) is generally referred to as B6, and it helps you use carbs that your body has stored. This vitamin not only helps to energize you, but makes more red blood cells that your body needs.

Biotin (B7) helps you metabolize fatty acids. Like many B vitamins, it also helps you process energy. It is found in many foods such as eggs, soybeans, and fish. When you are deficient in this vitamin, you may feel depressed, have muscle pain, and experience a reduced appetite.

Folate (B9) is found in fortified cereals, dark green vegetables, black-eyed peas, chickpeas, citrus fruits, and melons. This vitamin helps keep your red blood cell levels where they need to be. It also aids in protein metabolization and cell division. Without this vitamin, you may have increased odds of heart attack, stroke, or cancer. You may also have heartburn and diarrhea.

Cobalamin (B12) is found in animal products like eggs, meat, and dairy. It is also in fortified cereals. B12 is a critical vitamin as it keeps your brain and nervous system running, while also helping your red blood cells form. Vegans and some vegetarians may need to turn to supplements to ensure that they are getting B12 in their diets. Those who are deficient may feel exhausted and have nerve degeneration, which can culminate in paralysis.

Vitamin C (ascorbic acid) is known mostly for being in foods such as citrus fruits, but it can also be found in dark green vegetables and tropical fruits like mangoes, strawberries, cantaloupes, or papayas. This vitamin helps your body create collagen, which helps heal injuries and maintain bone strength. It also helps you absorb iron while working as an antioxidant that allows you to be more impervious to infections. The deficiency of this vitamin is called scurvy, which is notorious for impacting sailors in the 1700s who did not have proper nutrition while away at sea. Scurvy can cause emotional effects, such as depression and hysteria. It can also cause dental issues, increased odds of infection, impaired wound healing, and muscular problems.

Back to Basics – The Five Food Groups

Micronutrients should be consumed every day. If you make sure to have fruit and vegetables of varied types with your meals, you'll get most of the nutrients you need. Doing so makes it easier not to binge, and you'll feel a lot better.

Vegetables

Vegetables are one of the most important parts of your diet. They contain a high number of nutrients, but they are low-calorie options. You should have around two and a half cups of vegetables a day. Mix up the kinds of vegetables you eat because the more kinds you eat, the more diverse nutrients you will get from what you are eating. Unfortunately, most Americans do not get the required amount of vegetables.

Dark green vegetables and cruciferous vegetables are some of the most nutrient-dense vegetables. In this group, you have vegetables like broccoli, spinach, kale sugar snap peas, cauliflower, lettuce, and cabbage. Red and orange vegetables also are packed with nutrients and include peppers, tomatoes, carrots, and sweet potatoes, while starchy vegetables are more caloric and include potatoes, peas, and corn. Beans and legumes are sometimes categorized as vegetables, but they may also be called proteins. These beans and legumes include black beans, chickpeas, black-eyed peas, and lentils.

Use vegetables in your diet in creative ways. Cook them or eat them raw. Whatever you do, adding some more vegetables won't hurt, and it's hard to eat too many of this food group. Eating vegetables is not only a great way to make you feel full, which will help you not binge, but vegetables have also been shown to reduce people's risks of having heart disease.

Fruits

Fruits are a great, sweet choice to make you feel satisfied with your meal long after it has finished. Apples, for example, have been shown to have great health benefits. Apples, like many fruits, are high in fiber, which can make you feel satiated (more on that soon), and studies have shown that people who ate apples before their meals ate fewer calories. Apples have also been linked to reduced chances of stroke, lower cholesterol, and could even prevent cancer. Apples are just one of the many amazing fruits that can change your life.

According to the USDA, there are two subgroups within the fruit food group: whole fruit and fruit juice. It's preferable to eat whole fruits rather than fruit juice. Fruit juice may not have as many nutrients. Additionally, some fruit juices have a lot of added sugar, so if you opt to have fruit juice, try juices that are 100% fruit juice. You probably know many examples of fruits, but just to be thorough, fruit includes apples, mangos, grapefruits, raisins, and melons.

You should aim to have around two cups of fruit a day (one apple, as a reference, is about one and a half cups). While fruit does have sugar, it is a good natural sugar that doesn't have the same energy spike and crash of the sugars you see in sweets.

Grains

In your diet, you should aim to have about six ounces of grains per day. Grains can taste very satisfying and help satiate you. There are two groups of grains: whole grains and refined grains. Whole grains are grains that have the bran and germ of the grain intact while refined grains removed those two parts, leaving only the endosperm. The germ and the bran contain nutrients like B vitamins, fiber, and minerals; thus, by eliminating parts of the grain kernel, refined grains do not do as much for you nutritionally. The endosperm primarily contains just protein and carbs. Whole grains include whole-wheat bread, popcorn, oatmeal, and brown rice, while refined grains refer to white bread, pretzels, normal pasta, and grits.

Proteins

You already know how important proteins are, so much so that they are their own food group. Eggs and meat are a great source of protein. It can be found in nuts, soy, and seeds as well. Generally, people need around five and a half ounces of protein per day. Nutrition experts recommend that you have a variety of proteins in your diet.

Dairy

Finally, the last food group is dairy. This group includes milk, cheese, and yogurt. It's recommended that you choose low fat or fat-free dairy products whenever possible and that you have three cups of dairy per day. You may use dairy substitutions to get similar benefits (such as nut milk or soy milk).

The Dangers of "Bad" Foods & How They Affect You

Do You Eat "Bad" Foods?

With thousands of articles talking about foods that you should never eat, it can be confusing to figure out what foods are good for you. It's natural to want to classify foods as bad or good because doing so helps you feel less lost when it comes to your nutrition. By labeling foods good and bad, though, you start to employ black and white thinking. Accordingly, you start to categorize foods as things you should eat and things you shouldn't eat with no moderation. This mindset sets you up to binge because it makes you feel deprived. It's time to consider that you may demonize certain foods that don't deserve to be demonized. Now that you know more about nutrition, it should be clear that foods aren't bad or good; they're just different.

Ask yourself if there are foods that you put off limits and examine why you put them off-limits. Do certain foods always lead to a binge? Do you have "binge" foods versus "diet" foods? Are you scared that certain foods would cause weight gain? Identify why you judge foods as bad, and now, let me debunk why those foods aren't bad.

"Bad" Foods Lead to Restriction

The Minnesota Starvation Experiment expertly shows the impacts of restriction on eating behaviors. In November 1944, the University of Minnesota had thirty-six men, who were conscientious objectors to the war, take part in a thirteen-month experiment. These men were first put through a control period in which they were eating a normal amount of food, then a period in which the men were in a state of semi-starvation. The experiment concluded by observing their recovery period in which they increased their calorie intake. Scientists had wanted to also include a phase of starvation, but they could not continue with the experiment because even with a diet that was only restricted down to 1600 calories, the men faced severe psychological ramifications such as becoming suicidal, causing researchers to have to stop the experiment before they could study the full effects of starvation.

The results of this experiment were shocking and became foundational in the understanding of eating disorders. Even with just semi-starvation, the men's psychological states shifted drastically. Some men became despondent, while others became indifferent. Many were moody. They also experienced physical weakness, lowered body temperatures, and slower heart rates. Even their sex drive decreased because of being hungry. Some men were driven to the point of madness. More importantly, men became obsessed with food. They'd think about it even when they weren't at meals and talk about food during much of their free time. They dreamt about food and fantasized about it. They chewed a lot of gum to get the sensation of eating. Some even began to smoke more. They became more detached from social settings, and at mealtimes, they'd become protective over their food. They were starving and setting themselves up for extreme food behaviors when they finally could normally eat again.

As the men returned to normal eating, they became prone to binging. They'd eat what would be several normal meals at one time, causing stomach pain and headaches. During the refeeding process, many binge ate, and some would even purge the food they'd eaten in various ways. They felt ravenous, and they had increased concerns about their bodies. They didn't like to discard any food during refeeding, even if they were full. Many men felt emotionally worse during the refeeding, and they only seemed to feel positive when they talked about food, hunger, or even their weight. Further, some would go to desperate measures to get more food and would even look through the garbage for something to eat because they felt so exorbitantly hungry. Even after months of being able to eat sufficient levels of food, participants carried on their refeeding behaviors, showing the long-lasting impacts of deprivation.

Many diets endorse calorie counts that are equal to low semi-starvation numbers that the men in this experiment had to stuck to, so if you're choosing to utilize those fad diets, you are probably not getting the food you need to feel mentally okay. If any of the behaviors or side-effects experienced by men in the Minnesota Starvation Experiment sound familiar, you are probably in a binge-restriction cycle, and it's not a healthy place to be. You'll never lose weight using that method as much as you may want to, and you will never feel at peace with food.

You need to keep in mind that physiological and psychological restriction each have the same influences on your brain. Whether you physically are restricting or are just mentally restricting, you are *still restricting.* Just the act of thinking that you need to be dieting can cause you to feel deprived, which will result in your brain becoming fixated on the things you tell yourself are "bad." Calling foods bad foods puts you in the mindset of restriction, which will lead to your binge eating behavior when you allow yourself to eat again.

Restriction Leads to Binging

Binge eating is commonly caused by a restriction of some sort. Maybe the restriction wasn't your choice, such as in instances of food insecurity caused by poverty. Unfortunately, the amount of people who have food insecurity is up to fifteen percent, and nearly twenty-five million Americans live in food deserts, meaning food is harder to access because food stores are at least a mile away. Thus, economic factors can also make people feel deprived and be more likely to binge. Psychological deprivation often plays a role as well. In either scenario, when people feel like they are being deprived of food, they start to fixate on food like the men in the starvation experiment. When they finally allow themselves to eat a normal meal, they cannot stop eating because their bodies want to stock up on energy while they can.

Too many people follow a binge restriction cycle. The cycle usually starts with dieting. A person will limit their intake in hopes of getting healthier or losing weight. This restriction will then cause mental turmoil. You will start to crave all the foods that you can't have and be extra ravenous because you feel hungry. Then, to relieve the tension from not eating and alleviate the obsession, you will binge, and it may start as just one meal, but you will decide that since you are already "ruining" your diet that you might as well eat everything you didn't allow yourself to. You end up making your "cheat meal" count to the fullest before you try dieting again. After your binge, you will probably feel guilty for your behavior, which will make you feel insecure and worthless. Those with eating disorders such as bulimia may resort to actions such as the use of a laxative, exercise, or vomiting. The guilty feelings then lead people back into restricting again, making the binge-restrict cycle start anew.

The binge-restrict cycle ultimately doesn't do anyone any good. You always start right back where you started and are filled with guilty feelings. This process is driven by black and white thinking that perpetrates that there are bad foods and good foods. To get better, you need to break those barriers.

Food isn't Bad or Good… It Just Is

While foods have different nutritional levels and it is good for your body to have nutrient-dense food, having the occasional piece of bacon or glass of full-fat milk isn't going to kill you. Food should be joyful, and while I want you to start choosing healthy foods just because they'll make you feel more energized and improve the overall condition of your body, I don't want you to eliminate anything. All the rhetoric about cutting foods from your diet is unhealthy. Some people even suggest cutting great dietary sources like wheat! Of course, it would make sense to avoid foods that you are intolerant too, and many people are intolerant to milk and gluten, but don't eliminate anything just because someone told you it was unhealthy. You need food to live, and it is always okay to eat it if you're hungry and remember that eating bad foods sometimes is much better than not allowing yourself to eat. Your body needs energy primarily to complete the most basic functions. Therefore, consider how much nutrition the foods you're eating have, but don't classify foods into good and bad.

How to Respond to Emotional Eating With Healthy Options

Emotional eating can feel out of your control, but you can take steps to remedy this lack of control by understanding why you emotionally eat and how to choose healthier options. It's not easier to address your emotional eating because you've probably become so used to it that you've forgotten the root causes. However, when you put your emotional eating under the microscope, you should be able to find some enlightening patterns, which you can use to then make changes.

Emotional eating is your tendency to respond to your feelings by eating food instead of addressing your feelings. Thus, you need to know what triggers your emotional eating. Log in your journal times when you feel like eating and what emotions you're feeling during those times. It's good to know what feeling makes you binge because, with this knowledge, you can resist the binge and seek out healthier options when you know you're being tempted by emotional hunger rather than physical hunger. Some of the common causes are boredom, stress, anxiety, and bottled up emotions.

Be able to determine what is emotional hunger and what is physical hunger. Emotional hunger will often be triggered instantaneously by a negative feeling or even a good feeling while physical hunger will happen in gradients. You'll start feeling slight physical hunger before it hits you full force. Emotional hunger will also be linked to comfort foods that you turn to when you're feeling upset. Furthermore, emotional hunger doesn't stop when your stomach is full, while physical hunger does have an end. Know the differences between these two hungers to have better control over your eating.

Learn to enjoy treats. I always used to shame myself for having sweets or junk food. I told myself that I was too fat to have those things. As a result, I'd feel even worse about myself and eat even more than I would have just to fill that emotional hole in my stomach. When you have ice cream or other treats, savor them. Don't gulp them down in one bite. Take your time and appreciate the goodness you are eating.

Have snacks with you whenever you can. That way, if you start to feel hungry, you can tend to your hunger before it gets ravenous. When you're going to work, for example, don't just pack a lunch. Have a couple of snacks handy so that when you get home, you feel well-nourished and don't want to eat everything in your pantry. Avoid that feeling of deprivation altogether so that you can more easily handle recovery from binge eating.

Talk to yourself with kindness rather than with negativity. Using positive self-talk can go a long way in helping to tame your emotional eating. Too many people degrade themselves and have a constant loop of negative self-talk. You don't need to be your own worst enemy. Be kind to yourself and give yourself the encouragement and support that you need to thrive.

Go for a walk. Walking is great for your cardiovascular health, and it can be a meditative experience. Plus, it is not too taxing on your body. You can do something as simple as walking around your neighborhood or even just walk around your house for a while. I prefer nature walks, but wherever you walk, is up to you. Walking is one of my favorite activities when I'm feeling overwhelmed by emotions because it helps me slow my brain and think my actions through. It's worth a try for you too.

Meditation can be an ideal way to help you work through negative emotions and get back in touch with your body. Take some time to close your eyes, focus on your breathing, and become one with your body. You can use guided meditation video or audio, but the process of merely sitting down and breathing counts as meditation. It only takes five minutes a day to put you in a good headspace.

Find a way to relax that you can turn to nourish your feelings. Embrace your feelings rather than running away from them. Hobbies can be great ways to channel your feelings into something constructive. Creative activities like fiction writing or constructing models can let you work through your feelings while making you feel like a success rather than failure.

Dance around your house to your favorite song. This is a simple task, but it can make a stark difference. Play music you like and let your body sway to the music. Music and dancing can send feel-good chemicals through your body and be a good outlet for many people. You don't have to be a great dancer to move or even have rhythm. Just enjoy the sound and the motion, and you are doing it exactly right.

Talk to a loved one. Your friends and family probably want to do whatever they can to make sure that you are happy and healthy. Let them help! Be sure to set boundaries so that they don't add more stress to your life but call a friend when you are feeling emotional or send a text to your mom. Communicating with others is a great way to stop a binge because binges are secretive and isolating.

Find a professional to talk to when all else fails. It's okay to need more help. Many people may need a neutral party to talk about their issues and to help them curb emotional eating. There's nothing wrong with needing a boost from a profession. I saw a therapist when my binge eating was at its worst, and she helped me see patterns and behaviors that would have taken me much longer to notice, and I still seek treatment if I am struggling, though not as often.

By choosing healthier practices over emotional eating, you can learn to stop binging forever. It doesn't take major changes in your life to make the necessary swaps either. It's most important that you are willing to leave dieting behind and ready to choose enriching activities.

Chapter 4:
Create a Winning Strategy to Curb Overeating

Reduce Stress & Anxiety – Choose to Rest & Relax

Reducing stress and anxiety is important because stress and anxiety make you more likely to binge. When stressed or anxious, people are more likely to choose high-fat foods. According to the American Psychological Association, thirty-eight percent of Americans have reported eating too much because of stress. Half of these people said that they were overeating every week or more frequently. Without a doubt, ongoing stress influences the behaviors of many people. Further, your body is more likely to store fat when you are stressed. It's easier to let emotional eating overtake you when you feel that worried feeling in the pit of your stomach. Thus, taking care of your stress is one of the best ways to take care of your binge eating. Here are some ways in which you can choose to rest and relax rather than letting the chaos of your life drive you.

Avoid pushing yourself too hard. Many overachievers tend to want perfection from every area of their lives. I used to beat myself up over getting a ninety-nine on a test simply because I used academic achievement to alleviate the overall anxiety that I felt. We all want to succeed, and there's nothing wrong with ambition, but if you push yourself past what you can feasibly do and expect yourself to never mess up, you're in for a lifetime of worry. The more you try to control things you can't control, the less in control you'll have, so stop trying to dictate everything that happens in your life and learn to live with the uncertainty.

One of the best things that I did to alleviate my stress is I bought a stress ball. It's a little step to make your anxiety better, but it made a huge difference. You can get them for just a few dollars, and whenever you're starting to feel overwhelmed, you can squeeze them and let out some of the tension in your body. I still keep one beside me when I'm working or feeling otherwise anxious. Whenever a surge of anxiety strikes, I can squeeze my worry away.

Having a pet can be another great way to reduce stress. While pets can cause stress of their own for some people (especially if you have a brand new puppy that you have to train), animals are generally therapeutic. Physical touch can help alleviate stress (including human to human touch), so animals can provide a connection to another living creature that feels good. Petting your cat or dog can make you calm down, and having to care for a pet can make you focus on the needs of another being rather than worrying about everything else in life. My cat, Pearl, always makes me feel calmer (even when she's not in an affectionate mood), and just having her around makes me feel less lonely when my husband isn't home.

Disconnect from technology. If you're finding yourself getting too emotionally connected to your phone, put it away for a while. You don't need to be constantly checking in with work while you are at home. It's okay to need time away, and it's okay to put your phone on do not disturb. If you get text messages, it's okay not to answer right away. Sometimes, you need distance from the technology in your life that so distracts you and piles on even more stress. Technology can feel stressfully inescapable, but always remember that you choose when to turn your devices on.

If you do choose to use technology to relax, use it wisely. Social media, for example, is probably not the best idea because it can often cause you to compare yourself to others, which might make you feel even more stressed. Watching a fun comedy or reading a book on your ebook reader may be a great method to relax, but make sure you're not constantly checking your work email as you engage in these activities. The goal is to keep work at work and your personal life personal. By having some degree of separation, you can find spaces in which you can relax so that stress doesn't always loom.

Eat foods rich in potassium. While all nutrients are important, potassium especially can help relieve stress. Foods like bananas or potatoes can help normalize your blood pressure and make you feel more energized. Research has shown that potassium can ameliorate the health risks of stress, such as heart attack or stroke. Thus, while it may seem contrary for a binge eater to use food to relax, staying well-nourished can help your stress levels tremendously.

Listen to music. Any kind of music will help reduce stress, but classical music is known to cause extra significant changes. Whatever music you choose will send dopamine and other feel-good chemicals through your body. Play songs you love, and don't be afraid to sing along. Music can allow you time to escape your worries and have fun. Going to concerts is another suggestion that might help. Live music not only makes you feel good, but it makes you feel like you are part of a moment.

Take a trip. Vacations give you a chance to disconnect from your responsibilities—even just a weekend trip to somewhere close by can make you feel better. When you take a trip, you get to escape from your real life. You get to do things that you want to do rather than things that you feel like you have to do. Go to places that make you feel inner peace. I love weekend trips to my favorite Rhode Island beach, especially when it's first starting to get chilly in the fall. When I stand in front of the beautiful ocean with fog hanging over the water and sand, I can't help but feel I'm in a happier place. Find spaces that make you feel that same way.

Organize your life. Take control of things that you can control rather than worrying about what you can't. Most of what you worry about is out of your control, and that's why you worry about it. It is important to find projects that you have actual control over. You can easily organize your desk or sort through your junk drawer. By taking charge of disorganized spaces, you are defeating chaos, which feels incredibly cathartic. Focus on what you can do because anything else isn't worth your time.

Try crafting. Activities like cross-stitching, crocheting, or knitting can help release some of your anxiety. Plus, crafting will give you a chance to make some cool stuff that you can feel proud of. There's a craft out there for everyone; you just have to find it. When I decided to stop binging, I resumed knitting after years of not doing it, and it felt great to bring that hobby back into my life. Plus, it gave me a way to focus my brain without having to think too hard about all the things that were worrying me.

Start an herb garden or plant other plants that you love. Herbs are good for the air in your house and are purifying, but many also have properties that alleviate stress and anxiety. Researchers have discovered that being close to plants can help you relax. Research from Washington State University shows that stressed people experienced a drop in blood pressure when near plants. Some commonly used herbs to reduce stress are lavender, chamomile, and jasmine. If you don't want to tend to plants, getting a candle, or even just having tea can have a good impact.

Do things for yourself. This suggestion seems a little bit "duh," but doing things for yourself is a powerful statement to your body. Your brain will get the message that it should relax when you treat yourself gently. Take a bath, go to the spa for a day, or take charge of your skincare regime. Whatever it is that you consider self-care, do that. Treat your body with the attention it deserves and reassure it that it doesn't have to worry.

An easy act you can do to relieve stress is chew gum. One Australian study in 2008 showed that chewing gum could lower cortisol in your saliva, which is a stress hormone. Plus, gum can give you the sensation of eating, which is helpful for those of us who like to eat to distract us from our woes.

Make sure you are taking deep breaths. We all need to breathe, and we do it naturally, but our breaths can become shallow when we are stressed, so be sure to make the effort to take especially deep breaths when you are feeling stressed or anxious. Calming breaths can help tame your body's reactions to worry and make you feel better in the process.

Laugh a lot. Laughter has been found to have many health benefits. Not only does it lower stress hormones, but it can also increase good cholesterol levels. Laughing also allows you to fake it until you make it. Maybe you don't feel happy, but by laughing, you will start to feel happy the more you laugh. Watch comedies, talk to a funny friend, browse memes on the internet. Find ways to laugh even if you're feeling awful because the adage that laughter is the best medicine is accurate.

Become Friends With Fiber & Protein

As you know, diet is vital to being able to stop binge eating. The foods you eat can help you curb your overeating, but I want you to focus on fiber and protein. These are some of the foods that will make you feel the most satiated and therefore make you less likely to binge. Fiber and protein should become good friends of yours going forward because they will set you up for success in ways that other foods don't.

Fiber

Fiber is often underestimated by people in how important it is, but those who have a lack of fiber probably aren't feeling as great as they could be. Plus, those who don't have enough fiber may have bowel issues and satiety issues, meaning that adding some more fiber to your diet can change the way you eat and digest food.

Fiber is a type of carb, but it is not one that can be digested by your body, meaning that calories from fiber do not get used for energy. Usually, it's recommended that people have twenty-five to thirty-eight grams of fiber per day, but this number varies based on your size and metabolism. There are two types of fiber that you need to be aware of. They are both important, but they are processed differently by your body and are used for distinct functions. The two types are insoluble fiber and soluble fiber. Soluble fiber can be dissolved by water. It can also be metabolized as it goes through your digestive system. Insoluble fiber does not dissolve in water.

Another perk that fiber has is that it feeds your gut floras, which are good bacteria in your gut that help with various functions that your body couldn't otherwise do. These floras reside in your digestive tract, and they help control your blood sugar, weight, immune system, and they even have a part in brain operations. Trillions of bacteria are in your gut, and they all have unique purposes. Your body isn't able to digest fiber, but the bacteria can digest fiber to use it for better purposes!

Fiber takes up more room in your stomach, which means that whenever you eat fiber, you will feel fuller. Thus, just a little bit of fiber can go along way. Fiber is not the kind of food that you'd want to binge on because it would leave you in pain. When eating fiber, you are more likely to feel satisfied with a modest portion.

Research has shown that having ample fiber in your diet makes you eat less during your meal. Even though fibrous foods are low in calories and full of water, they make people feel more satiated. Apples, as we've discussed, cause people to eat less during meals. This impact has been found in other foods like lettuce as well. In studies of obese women, eating foods that have a lot of fiber resulted in the women feeling less hungry than when they had foods that had a lot of fat.

Be sure to gradually add fiber to your diet. If you increase your fiber levels too quickly, you will have gut pain and bowel issues that will make you uncomfortable. Because of the function of fiber and how bacteria eats it, you may have gassiness if you increase fiber too quickly. If you take your time introducing fiber, this will not be as much of a problem, so try to incrementally add more fiber into your diet until you have the required amount. This is not something that you should try to fix overnight, and your body will have to get used to increased levels of fiber.

Whole foods are often high in fiber. Try to eat many fruits and vegetables, which are low-calorie options that are packed with fiber. Do not remove the skins of fruits whenever possible because the skins often contain the fiber you need. Additionally, you can incorporate whole grains for improved gut function and satiety.

Without fiber, your digestive system simply won't thrive. Those who don't have enough fiber may have stomach discomfort and constipation, which no one wants. The research has long shown that adding more fiber to your diet can make you healthier. Plus, fiber has a myriad of health benefits that allow you to stay full longer without having to eat more food. A companion nutrient of fiber is protein, which has its own abilities that will help you stop binging and only eat as much food as you need.

Protein

We've already talked a lot about protein, but it deserves an extra spotlight because changing my relationship with protein helped me change my life. I'd never been much of a protein eater before. I'm a vegetarian, so I have to think outside the box when it comes to protein and ensure that I am getting all the amino acids I need. Nevertheless, when I started adding more proteins to my diet, I felt tangible changes. I had fewer thoughts of binging, and I didn't feel as though I had to eat so much. While my evidence is anecdotal, scientific studies have shown how helpful protein can be.

One clinical trial by Latner and Wilson from the International Journal of eating Disorders studied the impacts fo protein in women with bulimia nervous or BED, both conditions characterized by binge eating. The women were split into groups and given high-protein or high-carbohydrate foods three times a day over two-week timeframes. Patients who ate the high protein meals were less likely to binge than those who had lots of carbs or the base groups. Those who had the protein only binged, on average, just over one time a week while those in the control group binged around three times a week. Furthermore, those who had protein ate less food at mealtimes and said that not only were they fuller, but they had less hunger as well.

Protein is also good because it takes more energy to digest it compared to other macronutrients. Thus, it takes more for your body to digest protein, which means that increased levels of protein will stay in your system longer while carbs and fats won't be as sustainable. Protein will leave you very satiated, and amino acids found in protein let your body know that you are eating food. It tells the hypothalamus gland, which controls your appetite, that you're not starving.

Another positive aspect of protein is that it encourages fat loss. Instead of losing muscle, having more protein will make it more likely that you lose fat. Those looking to build strength will, therefore, benefit from protein intake without having to use means of restriction to improve their health. While weight loss shouldn't be the goal, protein can help with weight management for those who have had issues with fluctuating weight.

Create a Plan That Helps You Achieve Your Goals

Why You Need to Plan

A plan gives you direction and tells you what to focus on. You have to decide where you want to go with your plan and how you want to get there. Your plan is like a GPS; it tells you where to go on your journey as you steer yourself through the terrain presented to you. You have to fill in what stops you want to make along the way, but your plan will connect the dots for you so that you don't get lost as you get more into your journey.

Planning makes it easier to decide under pressure. When you have a plan, you have the focus you need to make decisions even under stress. You'll be able to choose a healthy snack right now over binging later with a plan. Planning gives you security because it reassures that you can handle your situation no matter how difficult it becomes.

Further, plans save you time. You have less to figure out along the way if you already have a good idea of what you want. You might as well determine what you want before you try to go for it. Otherwise, you'll waste time aimlessly wandering when you could be making strides to ending your binging for good.

How to Create a Good Plan

Decide what goals are most important to you. Also, create mile-markers along the way. If you want to stop binging by Christmas, write that goal down, but also have quantifiable mile-markers along the way. For example, say that you aim to cut down your binging by half midway to Christmas. Your goals can be customized to your interests and how quickly you can reasonably see progress. Be sure, however, that you're not trying to get from point A to point Z without any in-between goals or milestones.

Let your plan have flexibility. Too much rigidness puts you right back into an unhealthy mindset. Journeys often come with detours, but just like a GPS, be able to recalculate your direction and adapt to the terrain you're facing in the present. We cannot predict the future, so things happen, and plans change. Thus, allow your plan to be dynamic. Don't be so set on a specific path that you refuse to find new paths that might work better.

Acknowledge what you are good at and what you are not so good at so that you can react accordingly. Utilize your strong areas in your plan to undermine the areas in which you are not so good. Maybe you're good at resisting binging around other people but binge a lot during the holidays. In this case, you could plan to be around a lot of people during the holidays and make sure that you're never left alone for too long.

Let mealtimes be joyful but focus on nourishment over emotional hunger. Make sure your plan includes all the nutrients you need and make sure that it accounts for the joy that hunger can give you. Don't cancel Thanksgiving dinner because you're afraid that it will ruin your progress. Work it into your plan and learn to live with it.

Be realistic with yourself. Know that sticking to the plan won't always be easy, so don't expect your plan to unfold faster than is logical. Know yourself and use your past experiences to judge what your limits are and how much you can accomplish in a certain amount of time. Don't aim to end binging eating for good tomorrow with no looking back. You'll face a few steps forward, but you will also take a few steps back sometimes. That's part of progress.

Stop the Yo-Yo Diet & Create Healthy Habits

Yo-Yo Dieting, Oh No!

Yo-yo dieting refers to weight-cycling, which is the process of losing and gaining the same weight. It can be seen in many bingers who go between restricting and binging. While it may seem harmless, it can be bad for your health. Not only does it lead to a more weight gain in the long term, it also often causes a higher body fat percentage and loss of muscle. It can also contribute to conditions like type two diabetes and liver issues because yo-yo dieting can cause you to have a fatty liver—which causes increased blood pressure and higher odds of heart disease. In general, yo-yo dieting makes you feel frustrated and worthless, and the research suggests that weight-cycling is more unhealthy than being overweight. Yo-yo dieting will never give you any satisfaction, so stop the fad diets, stop trying to lose weight, and start making long-term changes that will leave you feeling better about yourself forever.

Create Healthy Habits

Healthy habits are one of the best ways to ensure that you stop binging. If you're able to incorporate some of these habits into your daily life, your body will not feel the same temptation to binge, and your body will thank you for showing it TLC.

Habit 1. Drink more water. You may mistake hunger for needing water, so be sure to keep yourself hydrated. Studies show that people who have water with meals tend to eat less. Furthermore, they feel less hungry at the end of their meals. Carry a water bottle around with you so that you can drink whenever you are thirsty.

Habit 2. Consistently eat meals. Skipping meals is not something that I want you even to consider. I know that diet culture has programmed you into thinking that it's normal to skip meals or replace meals with things like juices, but that's not acceptable. Skipping meals will only make you hungry, and I don't want you to feel hungry. I want you to tend to your body and feel full.

Habit 3. Use meal planning to figure out what you want to eat during the week. Studies have shown that people who use a meal plan tend to have better eating habits. All it takes is for you to take an hour or so each week to decide what you'll want to eat. Also, create a shopping list when you go to the grocery store. Doing so will help prevent you from buying foods you shouldn't.

Habit 4. Feel free to love food. Learn to love cooking it, and don't worry about being around it. Food is not the enemy here. It is good for your body and your mind. Let it do all the things that it should be doing. There's no point in fighting it.

Habit 5. Nourish yourself with things other than food. Focus on your personal relationships, your career, or your spiritual connections to improve your connection between your mind and your body. If you feel nourished in those areas, you will have less need to emotionally eat.

Habit 6. Use your food journal. Write in it every day. This is one of the healthiest habits you can engage in, especially when you're starting your journey to end binging. Remaining vigilant about your eating habits will allow you to better understand your bodily needs and emotional needs when it comes to food.

Habit 7. Honor your cravings. Get in the habit of telling yourself that you can have the foods you crave. Don't get caught up in a restriction mentality. Eat cake at your niece's birthday party without guilt!

Habit 8. Don't let yourself walk away from traditions. You can still have food traditions that remind you of your childhood. Just like you shouldn't deprive yourself of any food, you shouldn't neglect your traditions either because they are part of who you are.

Habit 9. Don't look at food as a punishment or a reward. It's just food. You can enjoy it, but you get to eat it whether you've done well or have failed. You always deserve food, and it's not reflective of how successful you are.

Chapter 5:
Change The Way You Eat…Permanently

A Look at Healthy Meals, Snacks, and Beyond!

Healthy Meals

Healthy meals will include items from all five food groups, so you can mix and match as you please, but here are some options for your consideration.

For all of you who don't eat meat, try a brown rice bowl for your meal. For protein (and grains), you can pair black beans with the rice. For your vegetables, you can add some peppers, tomatoes, and spinach. You can top it all off with some cheese to get your dairy requirement. For dessert, you can have some strawberries with whipped cream to fulfill your fruit requirement.

For you meat-eaters, you can have a healthier version of chicken parmesan. You can have grilled chicken sprinkled with sauce, tomatoes, and a sprinkle of cheese. For your sides, you can have whole grain pasta and steamed broccoli. For dessert, you can have a scoop of ice cream and add a banana to make a banana split. If you don't like any of that, there are plenty of swaps that you can make to include items that you do like. That's the joy of the food groups— you can combine them how you please.

Make an effort to research new dishes and try new food combinations that you've never tried before. Don't let yourself be too safe with what you eat. Some variety will keep you more satisfied than eating the same five things.

Healthy Snacks

There are lots of healthy snacks that can help keep you satiated and feeling good throughout the day. Find snacks that you like and keep your body going.

Nuts are one of the best snacks that you can have because they are very filling and packed with healthy fats. One of my favorite nuts is an almond because almonds taste great, have lots of protein and fiber, and they are easy to bring with me to work or other functions. They are a superfood, making them a great choice for anyone.

Having red bell pepper strips with avocado is another nutritious snack choice. This snack is less portable, but it too is filled with nutrients and healthy fats from the avocado. Moreover, red bell peppers fill you up without being too high in calories.

Apples and a nut butter of your choice are a sweet delicacy. Again, they are filled with fiber, and nut butter (such as almond butter or peanut butter) adds some protein. This snack is both satiating and feels like it's a special treat.

A final snack idea I'll give you is kale chips, which can feed your craving for something crunchy. Being a leafy green vegetable, kale is packed with nutrients and is full of fiber.

Ultimately, be creative with your snacks, but try to find ones that combine a couple of foods to add nutrients that will keep you full between meals.

Be Emotionally Well-Fed

Check-in with how you are feeling throughout your day so that you never starve your emotions of the attention that they need. Even when you are busy, you need to make time to check-in with yourself because if you don't, you'll find yourself being emotionally hungry. This will ultimately lead to a binge no matter how well you've been eating and physically nourishing yourself.

You cannot have full physical health if you are not mentally healthy. When you're not mentally healthy, all your bodily systems cannot work at peak function. Let yourself feel content with where you are right now so that you can enjoy your food without wanting to overindulge. This is key to defeating binge eating for good.

Get Up and Move – The Benefits of Exercise

Why Exercise?

Exercise may seem like a drag, and it can be arduous work, but it is good for you to get moving. The statistics on physical activity among adults show how inactive people have become. Shockingly, fewer than five percent of adults exercise daily. A hefty eighty percent of adults do not do enough strengthening or aerobic activity. Nearly thirteen percent of people without disabilities aren't active at all during the week. Thus, many people are not experiencing the immense benefits of working out. By adding a little bit of exercise each day, you can transform your life and your relationship to food.

Mood regulation is one significant effect of exercise. Exercise results in your body, releasing endorphins, which make you feel happier. Thus, exercise can help alleviate depression or anxiety. If you're an emotional eater, you know how much your mood can trigger your binging, so get in control of your mood by employing physical activity. To be happy, you must ensure that your body and mind are well taken care of, and exercise can help you do both.

Exercise has an impact on your physical health, of course. It lowers your blood pressure, and it reduces bad cholesterol. Those who exercise also experience better heart health and circulation. They are less likely to get type two diabetes. Exercise is also good for both your bone health and muscle health.

People who exercise sleep better according to research. When you sleep better, you eat better and are less stressed, making sleep directly and indirectly helpful to you—those who exercise sleep for longer and more thoroughly. When you don't get enough sleep, your body's hormones go out of whack. People who get less than seven hours of sleep per night may experience increased ghrelin levels and decreased leptin levels. Ghrelin is the hormone that makes you have an appetite while leptin tells you when you are full. Thus, people who don't get enough sleep not only tend to overeat, but they also tend to choose easy to prepare, high-fat foods that have little nutritional value and do not keep them satiated.

It may not seem like it, but physical activity can make you feel more energized rather than more tired. Those who exercise feel better able to move and accomplish daily life tasks. Moreover, people who are active live longer, and if that's not a good enough reason to get moving, I don't know what is.

Exercising just thirty minutes once a week can improve your binge eating. Doing exercise, no matter how old you are or how inactive, can set you up for a better future, and it's never too late to start, but don't keep waiting to work out. Do it as soon as you finish this book because it will help you make peace with the monster in your mind.

How to Get Moving

You need to get moving, but don't worry about getting moving in the "right" way. There's no wrong way to get moving as long as you are getting your body to be more active. The point is to be active, not to overburden yourself or hurt your body, so don't push yourself past your limits.

Head to the gym. While gyms aren't for everyone, they have a large amount of equipment and classes that you won't be able to find in your house. At a gym, you can get a variety of exercises for one consistent price. Many are open twenty-four seven, making them fairly convenient.

Find a workout buddy. When I started exercising, I was shy about going to the gym, so I asked my best friend if she would be interested in heading to the gym with me. We both wanted to get more active, so it worked out well for both of us. Having someone to get active with makes the experience markedly more enjoyable, and you can keep each other accountable so that you don't slack off.

Take an exercise class. Lots of gyms and studios have fun workout classes led by instructors. Yoga, pilates, Zumba, ballet barre, and other work out programs can get your blood pumping while still being fun. Many include dance elements and great music!

Go outdoors. Walking, hiking or biking are all some good options for both getting active and enjoying the great outdoors. If you have a pool in your yard or a local outdoor pool, swimming is a fantastic low-impact option for people looking to strengthen their bodies. Being outside feels meditative and less rigid than going to the gym for many people.

Workout at home. Whether you get equipment, use recorded workout programs, play fitness games, or even just walk up and down your steps, you can get an extensive workout at home.

Journal about your progress. Your fitness goals and progress reports have a place in your journal. Write down how much you move and what kind of exercises you do. Try to build up and improve your skillsets as you go. Write down things you want to be able to do with your body in the future and plan to work towards those goals.

Search the internet for workouts. There's plenty of workouts at the touch of your fingers, so don't be afraid to scour the internet for different programs that might meet your skills and fitness needs.

Get a personal trainer. If you're feeling a bit lost, it may help to have a personal trainer who can guide you about proper workout procedures and make sure that you don't hurt yourself by using certain equipment the wrong way.

Whatever it is that you do, make sure that you enjoy it. Working out won't always be pleasant, but it needs to make you feel satisfied and healthy.

With a Little Help From My Friends

You should get your friends involved in your process to end binge eating. Binge eating is such a solitary experience that working through it alone feels overwhelming. When my life was shrouded in secrecy, and even the closest people to me didn't realize what I was going through, I felt so depressed, and I wondered if I'd ever be motivated to get better.

Breakthrough your shame and tell friends what has been going on with you because sharing this awful experience will lift a weight from your shoulders, and your friendship will be better once you are honest. You'll be more vulnerable and share deep, important parts of yourself that you felt you needed to hide in the past.

Eat with friends. When I eat with friends, I'm distracted from the food in front of me, and while you may still feel urges to binge, it's much easier to stay on track when you're not eating alone. Plan to have as many meals as you can with other people. It may feel mortifying at first, or you may feel silly asking friends or loved ones to eat meals with you, but it does help.

Don't let your pride stand in the way of letting your friends do what they can to help you. Your loved ones want you to be happy and healthy, and their offers of help shouldn't be taken defensively. Be sure to tell them when they've stepped too far, but allow them to help when they can because you need their support.

Give your friends boundaries. Accepting help is wonderful, but we all have certain boundaries that we need to maintain, or else relationships start to crumble and feel toxic. Let them know things that trigger you and will only make you worse. Put your recovery first!

Spend more time with your friends. Being social is important to human well-being. Accordingly, the simple act of spending more time with people who you love can empower you and make you feel more comfortable in your own skin. When you spend time with your friends, focus on your relationships with those people rather than your relationship with food. Your friends deserve your attention too, so be there for them as much as they are there for you. Don't be scared to try new things with the people you love. Expand your boundaries and create new memories with your friends.

Ask your friends to hold you accountable, and keep them updated on your progress. Share the obstacles along with the successes. Let them know how you've been doing so that they can push you to continue to make progress. Never revert to being ashamed. Find at least one person who will listen to your struggles and celebrate your victories. You have a rocky path ahead of you, and sometimes, you'll fall, but you'll get to your destination with friends who are willing to pull you up.

Cut out any toxic friends. People who make you feel bad about yourself should have no place in your life. Losing friends is hard, and walking away from friendships takes courage, but sometimes doing so is vital. If people cannot accept you as you are, then they are not worth keeping around because they'll only cause you heartache.

Don't be afraid to ask for advice or your friend's open ear. If you need to talk, don't keep what you have to say bottled up. Writing your feelings down is helpful, but confessing them to a waiting ear can be even more cathartic. Be bold and talk about your emotions so that your feelings cannot get the best of you. Your friends might even give you some new insight that you never considered before, speeding up your recovery process substantially.

Value yourself as your friends value you. I used to always think my friends were too great to truly like someone like me. I figured that it was a fluke that they chose to hang out with me when I wasn't anyone special or cool, but the thing is that my friends *did* think that I was special and cool. They saw qualities about me that I couldn't see. Try to look at yourself from that perspective and realize that the negativity you have about yourself is not how other people look at you.

Your friends are some of the most important people in your life. They may even be like family to you. You've been through a lot together, I'm sure, and you can get through binge eating too. This is not a battle you have to fight alone. You have allies, and it's time to turn to them and let them into this part of your life.

Never Give Up, Never Surrender

Why You Should Persist

You need to persist through your recovery process even if it seems hard because recovering from your binge eating is going to change your entire future. You have two options. You can either continue your life as it is, or you can change. Persist past all the pain. Persist past all the cravings. Persist past all the slipups. Move past all the hardship, and you'll finally be free from binging your life away. Your future is in your hands, and the beautiful thing is that you're the one who defines what happens next. There's so much that you can't predict in your future, but no matter who you are, you can craft a future worth living.

How to Get Through Hardship

Believe in yourself. This is the most important thing that you can do. Don't doubt your ability to get through this. If you say that you will never stop binging, you will never stop binging. That's the bottom line. You become your inner dialogue, so starting telling yourself that you will succeed. Write it on sticky notes and repeat it to yourself each time you wake up, and each time you go to bed. Repeat after me, "I will succeed. I will be free from binge eating. I will be fully me, and I will not let my disorder control who I will be."

Know that obstacles aren't the death of progress. If you've abstained from binging for a week and then find yourself binging again, you don't have to keep binging. A slip up doesn't mean that you've failed at recovery. I cannot tell you how many times I slipped up and went back to binging. I'd go weeks or months without it, and then I'd find myself back to doing it again, but I didn't give up. I used those mistakes to make myself even more determined to get better. Be stubborn, and don't let obstacles define what will become of you.

Remember that as long as you are trying to get better then you *are* getting better. You are better than you were when you weren't trying to cure your disorder. You've already made substantial progress coming this far. The hardest part is admitting to yourself that you have a problem. All that's left is to fight for recovery and always keep your end goals in sight. Never forget why you are trying to get better. You're trying to save yourself from the misery of binging. You're doing your best, and you will find peace soon. Just hold on a little longer.

Don't forget that you're through the worst of your binging. If you're reading this book, you don't have to let your binge eating get worse. Your worst day can already be over, and from here, it will be uphill. Recovery is like a mountain range. You have ups and downs that you have to travel across, but you'll get better at managing the terrain, and you'll learn how to get yourself through the lows so that when the highs come, you can enjoy your breathtaking surroundings. As long as you are practicing recovery, you can never be kicked down forever, so get up on your feet, and let's go!

Living With the Long-Term Results

Changes That Last

If you want long-term results, you have to make changes that will last. Don't look at these changes as something you can stop once you finally stop binge eating. You have to continue these practices for the rest of your life. They will become more instinctual, but you'll never be able to go on a diet again because going on a diet would bring you right back where you started. You can't make losing weight your main purpose, either. If it happens, it happens, but it may not. Make peace with the fact that the number on the scale might not change (but your body certainly will when you stop binging).

Tell yourself that you can make lasting change. Self-doubt is only going to create a self-fulfilling prophecy. Believe in this process and give it your all. Adjust my recommendations to your specific needs, but let yourself give these steps and tools a valiant try because I guarantee that you won't be worse off for them.

Keep the person you want to be in mind, and know that there are lots of success stories. You can be that person who you're dreaming of being. It may take a lot of work to get there, but there is hope for you. Anyone who sets their mind to it can end the binge-restrict cycle.

How to Stick to a Plan

Sticking to a plan is hard for many people, but fear not, there are steps that you can take to ensure that you don't wander from your aspirations.

Write your plan down. Hopefully, you've already done this in the planning portion of the book. Mental health experts generally use the acronym S.M.A.R.T. to dictate what goals should look like: specific, measurable, achievable, realistic, and timely. Keep these terms in mind as you're trying to keep to your plan. Post sticky notes around your house to easily remember what you are working towards. The more you are exposed to your goals, the better your results will be. Don't just write them down, though, repeat your goals out loud because doing so will help your brain absorb your aspirations even more.

Don't do too much at once. Focus on one behavior that you need to change, and then once you accomplish that, work on others. Taking on too many behaviors at once will only overwhelm you. It's better to take your time to stop your binge eating than to rush through, so work on one issue at once and add more as you feel comfortable doing so.

Make manageable deadlines that make up smaller goals and build to your larger goal. Deadlines are good because they are quantifiable, but be careful not to make them too rigid. Furthermore, don't make your only deadlines long-term. Have milestones leading up to the longer-term deadlines. You should also note that deadlines aren't the end-all and be-all of success. If you miss a deadline, you can still succeed. Look at the deadlines as an ETA rather than as a time you need to be there. By doing this, you can take some of the pressure off, which will make it easier to reach your goals. You will progress at your own pace, but you can push yourself to move at your quickest rate.

Have a non-food related prize for when you reach your goals. This prize can be anything that you want. Maybe you want to buy new clothes, or maybe you want to buy your family a dog. Whatever it is that you want, reward yourself along the way. While you won't get instant gratification, you can still be gratified at various points in the process.

Hold yourself accountable for when you don't reach your goals. Don't look at mishaps as failures. Instead, see them as opportunities to do better. Whenever you miss your goal, it's a chance to learn and know what to do differently next time.

Conclusion

As our time together comes to a close, I want to review all the progress you've made during this book, and the lessons you've learned because believe it or not, the strides you've made are significant. The information you've read here will serve you for the rest of your life. I hope you can apply these lessons to yourself and find the freedom that you deserve. Progress may be slow, but it will come.

I've been free of binge eating for years, but it also took me years to get to this point, and even now, there are still days when I struggle. Food does not run my life. I am free, and I want more than anything for you to be free as well because no one deserves to live with the binge monster inside of them. Binge eating is a dark, lonely disorder, but it's not incurable.

You've gone to the root of your binge eating, and examined the personal and cultural aspects that may influence your binge eating. If you didn't know, you learned the difference between mere overeating and binge eating. You learned how prevalent food issues are in our culture and how these issues are influenced by societal, environmental, and biological factors. Hopefully, you realized that you are far from alone in your binge eating. Too often, binge eating is normalized or made into a joke on sitcoms, but it is a real issue that devastates lives and makes it hard for people to engage in regular activities, particularly ones that are related to food. Continue to dig into why you started binge eating and under what conditions you do it because these answers will guide you as you make recovery permanent.

You've discovered the joy of eating slowly and the importance of slowing down your rapid thoughts by journaling. You need to appreciate your food rather than stuffing it into your face as fast as possible. Slow eating allows you to be more mindful and keeps your hunger cue engaged, so you don't fill yourself past your limit. You've learned to resist the urge of instant gratification and to realize that you must wait for progress because it takes months or even years to improve your binge eating. Make incremental goals that power you through each day and motivate you to continue striving for your best. To stay mindful of your eating habits and your goals, you can use a food journal to track what you're eating and how you feel when you're eating it, among other aspirations such as exercise goals or food ideas. You've learned to listen to your hunger, both emotional and physical, which will benefit you in the rest of this process.

You've seen the power of nutrition and the types of foods that you should be eating to make sure your body feels nourished and doesn't want to binge. The urge to binge often biologically stems from being deprived. The Minnesota Starvation Experiment shows that people become obsessed with food even when only moderately deprived, leading to binging. Furthermore, dividing foods into the categories of good and bad can be equally dangerous because doing so creates a similar restriction mindest. It makes you feel deprived. Your body fears that it is going to starve, so it eats as much as it can. While foods aren't good or bad, you need to pay attention to what you are eating because certain foods are more satiating than others, and if you want your body to be satisfied, you need to get all your nutrients. Be sure to include all five food groups as well as the three main macronutrients and the micronutrients, which include vitamins and minerals, in your diet.

You've created a strategy to curb overeating and take back your body. Find ways to manage your stress. Don't let your emotions decide what you're going to eat. Take the power of your body back. Include more fiber and protein in your diet because they are good for digestion and satiation. Plus, they have a myriad of other health benefits that will boost your energy. Learn to plan for your future, including your goals and meals, and practice swapping emotional eating for healthier options that will give you the energy to get up and live your life.

You've learned how to manage your feelings and personal life in ways that aren't overeating; these skills will help you create long-term change and allow you to be free for the rest of your life. Be creative when including healthy meals, snacks, and emotional energy into your diet. Have fun trying new things and exploring healthy dishes. Another great way to manage your binge eating recovery is to get up and move. Incorporate more exercise into your life and have fun doing it. Further, don't handle your struggles alone. Invite friends into your personal life and allow them to help you get better. Don't let yourself give up on your progress. Believe in yourself so that you can live with the long-term results and never go back to how you were before. There's no time for turning back. Reach out for your future and take it.

In all these lessons, I have taught you why you are binge eating and how you can put an end to it without having to torture yourself with dieting or eating foods that you hate. I've shown that you can successfully eliminate binging while still being the person you've always been. My goal was never to change who you are but to allow that person to exist again after being suffocated by binge eating for so long because that person deserves to feel fully alive.

I appreciate you reaching the end of *Stop Binge Eating 101*, and I sincerely hope that it gave you the tools and information that you need to end your battle with binge eating forever.

What I need you to do now is to put this plan into action and finally free yourself from binge eating. There's no looking back. Don't wait until tomorrow to do it. Change your life right now, and if you don't take anything else away from this book, I want you to know that there's nothing to be ashamed of if you are a binge eater. Your dignity and worth as a person are not changed based on what you eat, and I hope you can love yourself and embrace the unique person who you are. Binging or not, you're still the same amazing person you have always been!

Intuitive Eating for Beginners

The Anti Diet Approach to Weight Loss and Disordered Eating

By

Monica E. Harris

INTUITIVE EATING FOR BEGINNERS
First Edition. July 29, 2020.
Copyright © 2020 Monica E. Harris

The data, depictions, events, descriptions, and all other information forthwith are considered to be true, fair, and accurate unless the work is expressly described as a work of fiction. Regardless of the nature of this work, the Publisher is exempt from any responsibility of actions taken by the reader in conjunction with this work. The Publisher acknowledges that the reader acts of their own accord and releases the author and Publisher of any responsibility for the observance of tips, advice, counsel, strategies, and techniques that may be offered in this volume.

Table of Contents

Introduction

For many years, I struggled with binge eating and found myself bouncing from diet to diet with little results. Like most women, I spent countless hours worried about my body image, all the while struggling to control my weight. Through the ups and downs, I found myself resorting to disordered eating, which didn't help my situation. In fact, it made it worse.

I felt stuck. Hopeless at the idea of ever being able to kick the habit and lose weight.

Chances are, you might relate to this feeling. You might be finding yourself at a crossroads with your weight, health or dieting in general. Worse yet, if you are like me, you may have found yourself having a rocky relationship with food.

If you are frustrated with dieting and unable to stop disordered eating, this book is written for you!

When I learned about the non-diet method of intuitive eating, a major shift occurred in my life. I saw diet culture as the enemy and found that my own connection to my body allowed me to open my eyes about how I ate. Over time, my thinking changed radically and my health improved as a result. This method has been proven to work for many people with different body types. And after reading this book, you can be one of those people too.

Intuitively eating is not a quick fix or a fad diet. It's a lifestyle and mindset that will benefit many aspects of your health. By following this non-diet method of intuitive eating, you will find numerous benefits including the following:

- Higher self-esteem
- Better body image
- More optimism
- Lower body mass indexes
- Higher HDL cholesterol levels
- Lower Triglyceride levels
- Lower rates of emotional eating
- Lower rates of disordered eating

According to scientists who published an article in the Journal of the Academy of Nutrition and Dietetics, this method of eating is proven to help people lose weight for good, and to maintain their healthy weight once they reach it. Also, this "non-diet" approach led to improvements in cholesterol levels.

Through reading this book, you will be sure to develop new perspectives on dieting and eating, along with new perspectives on exercise. You will also find new ways of looking at your body and the importance of loving yourself. This will ultimately lead you to gain a new lease on life. There has never been a better time to take your eating habits and your lifestyle into your own hands and change it for the better.

If you want to start feeling and living more optimally, the information in this book will help you do so.

This book will allow you to find a solution for your weight and eating struggles. I guarantee that it will exceed your expectations in terms of how it will change your mind forever. You will thank yourself for choosing this book as you move forward in your life.

Get ready to start your journey in the next chapter, where we will begin by looking at the theory of intuitive eating and how it can help change your life for the better.

Chapter 1: What is Intuitive Eating?

Let us start by looking at what exactly intuitive eating is, as well as a brief history of how this style of eating came about. This chapter will provide you with a solid foundation of knowledge on which to build your new lifestyle.

What Is Intuitive Eating?

Intuitive eating, at its core, is a style of eating that puts you in the driver's seat of your own life. The practice of intuitive eating encourages you to listen to your body. This, in turn, allows you to provide your body the foods it needs *when it needs them*.

Intuitive eating is different than a traditional diet. Instead of following a set of guidelines that tell you when and what to eat, you learn to listen to your body because it has all the answers.

Intuitive eating does not limit certain foods or require you to stick to restrictive meals exclusively, but instead encourages you to learn as much as you can about what your body is telling you in regards to its hunger and needs.

There are two main components to intuitive eating:

- Eat when you are hungry
- Stop eating when you are satiated

As odd as it may seem, humans are very far from this kind of eating in today's world. With so many diet trends and numerous "rules" for how you should and should not eat, it can be difficult to put these ideas aside and let your body do the talking.

The History Of Intuitive Eating

Though it may seem as though intuitive eating is a concept that has been around forever, it is a relatively new concept as far as modern eating styles go. The origins of intuitive eating are said to be dated to around 1978 when a book called "Fat is a Feminist Issue." was written. This book discussed many of the same types of ideas around eating, diet culture, and body image.

Similarly, in 1995, two women wrote a book about intuitive eating, which aimed to help women to achieve a better body image and experience less guilt around eating. This is when the term "Intuitive Eating" was first developed, and it has been used to describe this style of eating ever since.

While the beginnings of intuitive eating are rooted in feminism and the pressure that is put on women by diet culture, both men and women can benefit from it. It is a style of eating and living that is best for the human body in general.

What are the Rules of Intuitive Eating?

In this section, we are going to look at the foundational rules of intuitive eating. I will begin by explaining what these are, and then we will examine the best approach to take when it comes to making a change in your life, especially when this change is related to the way that you eat.

These rules serve to outline the philosophy of intuitive eating and how it can be employed in anybody's life. Over the next several chapters, we will look at many of these concepts and how they can help you gain a better understanding of intuitive eating.

Intuitive Eating Rule #1. Adhere To Your Hunger

In diet culture, hunger is seen as an enemy. However, when it comes to intuitive eating, hunger is not an enemy, but rather a source of valuable information for you regarding what your body is asking for and what it needs.

The main philosophy behind rule number one is: You must respect your hunger.

This means that you must respond when your body signals the need for nutrients and sustenance. If you don't acknowledge your hunger, you will likely wait until you are ravenous before eating. If this is the case, you will be much more likely to overeat. If instead you had trusted your hunger and eaten when you first became hungry, you would have eaten the right amount and been much less inclined to overeat. When you choose to adhere to your hunger and eat when your body tells you that it needs sustenance, you are much more likely to eat just the right amount, and you and your body will be satisfied rather than completely stuffed afterward.

You must reject feeling shameful and angry for being hungry and learn to feel happy that your body is telling you what it needs. Be thankful that you can provide it with nutrients for it to keep working hard for you!

Intuitive Eating Rule #2. Say No To The Diet Industry

At first glance, the diet industry may seem like it is concerned with helping people to improve their lives. However, this is not the case. In reality, the diet industry is concerned with making money.

The diet industry grows their revenue by convincing people that they should try a specific diet plan, followed by, another and another. People who fail to find results when following these diet plans will try many different diet trends, spending large amounts of money in the hopes of finding one that finally works.

The diet industry is also focused on making you feel like you are not perfect enough. Looking at your body from the perspective that it is not perfect will ultimately leave you feeling like a failure. Since you will never achieve perfection, you will never feel satisfaction from these diets. For this reason, you will forever be chasing the "right diet" when, in fact, there is no "right diet," there is only the best way that you can fuel your own personal body by giving it what it needs. This is where intuitive eating comes in.

When it comes to being healthy and taking good care of your body, intuitive eating is not a diet. It is instead a philosophy that aims to help you return to the traditional way that humans ate before diets were created.

To follow intuitive eating properly, you must acknowledge that the diet industry itself is harmful to you. You must begin to embrace that your own body holds the key to effectively losing weight.

Intuitive Eating Rule #3. Don't Restrict What You Eat

When trying to make a lifestyle change or trying to modify habits that are firmly ingrained in your day to day life, the approach you take will play a large part in whether you succeed or relapse. The basics of this principle will pave the way for you to start taking real action and start taking steps toward a new way of eating that will improve your life. This principle is all about not falling prey to restrictive eating.

Intuitive eating is a good choice for anyone, especially for those who prefer more flexibility when it comes to their eating time and those who do not want to restrict their meals at all. Humans should not be putting themselves through boot camp every time they feel hungry, and this method does not adhere to that type of mindset.

One of the reasons that intuitive eating is such a successful and cherished form of eating is that it allows the body to lead the mind in the right direction when it comes to seeking out its needs.

Paying attention to the messages your brain is sending your body and knowing how to deal with them is essential. For example, did you know that your cravings could be giving you much more information than you give them credit for? Below we will look at what your cravings could mean and why you should let your body guide your eating choices.

A craving is an intense longing for something (in this case food), that comes about strong and sudden.

In your case, that longing is probably for a certain food. When we have cravings for specific foods, it can mean more than what it seems. While you may chalk it up to simply being hungry, your cravings may instead be indicating a nutrient deficiency.

Why is this? A craving comes about because the body thinks that the nutrients it needs can be gained through eating a certain food. As a result, the body tells you that it wants that particular food. This is why a craving feels so urgent. The body is trying to help itself by telling you what to eat. But to us, this feels like an intense craving.

Sometimes the things we crave won't be the best way to get the vitamins or minerals that we need. Having the nutrients that you need in the right amount helps to regulate mood, hunger, and cravings. Thus, when one or more of these nutrients are low, it is hard for us to regulate our appetite and our cravings, and this is why we tend to long for foods that are not always the best ways to receive these nutrients. For this reason, understanding your cravings can help you give your body exactly what it needs.

- Chocolate And Magnesium

When we crave chocolate, this means our body is low in Magnesium. Dark chocolate naturally contains high levels of Magnesium.

When you are experiencing a craving for chocolate, it usually comes in the form of a craving for a doughnut or a chocolate bar. The problem with this, is that this form of chocolate contains high amounts of sugar, fat, and oil, and not enough magnesium to help your body combat this craving for good.

The next time you crave chocolate, keep in mind that it may be due to a magnesium deficiency. Other signs of a magnesium deficiency can include general sugar cravings, which explains why you crave sweets.

When your body consumes sugar, it must use magnesium in order to process it for digestion. For this reason, giving in to your cravings of sugar may actually end up further reducing your body's magnesium levels, which will send you into a cycle of more sugar cravings and an increasing level of magnesium deficiency.

Chocolate by itself is actually quite rich in nutrients. However, it is the actual pure cocoa that holds all of these nutrients. If you are going to eat chocolate to ease your sugar cravings and your need for magnesium, make sure that it is dark chocolate. To get the most nutrients possible, be sure that the dark chocolate you choose comes with at least 70% cocoa content. Cocoa contains high levels of magnesium, iron, fiber, and antioxidants. While you are getting your magnesium fix, you will also be getting your fill of other good nutrients that your body needs.

If you have low magnesium levels, there are many other ways you can replenish it. Eating nuts like almonds and cashews is a great choice as they are high in magnesium and may give your body exactly what it needs. If you crave chocolate, try eating these magnesium-rich foods at your next meal and your chocolate craving may just dissipate.

- Hydration

If you are craving juice or pop or other sugary drinks, consider that you might be dehydrated and, therefore, thirsty. Sometimes we see drinks in our fridge, and since we are thirsty, we want to reach for them. Sometimes, however, we are simply in need of water. After all, water is the best thing to quench your thirst.

The next time you are craving a sugary drink, try having a glass of water first, then wait a few minutes and see if you are still craving that Coca-Cola. You may not want it anymore once your thirst has been quenched.

- Salty Foods

If you are craving salty foods like chips or pizza, your body might be low in Sodium. We must be careful with this one as being low in sodium is quite rare given our modern diets. It could be, however, if you sweat a lot that this deficiency occurs. If this is the case, though, try reaching for something more natural like celery, milk, or even beets. While these may seem like odd sources of sodium as they don't taste particularly salty, these three foods contain natural sodium. They are also not nearly as bad for the body as fast foods are.

- Meat

If you are craving meat, you may feel like you want some fried chicken or a hot dog. This can indicate a deficit of iron or protein. The best sources of protein are chicken breast cooked in the oven, while iron is best received from spinach, oysters, or lentils. If you think you may not like these foods, there are many different ways to prepare them, and you can likely find a way that you enjoy. As long as they are not fried, this will be much better for you than a hot dog or fried chicken. The other way to get iron is from lean beef, which can be found in a lean steak.

Craving meat can also mean that you are lacking in vitamin b12. Vitamin B12 is found in meat and other animal products. Vitamin b12 helps the body to have a healthy bloodstream as well as a good memory. To get this, you want to eat good sources of organic meats as well as eggs and turkey.

- Calcium

If you find yourself craving cheese, it could be because of a Calcium deficit. To find out if this is the case, you need to try eating other foods that are rich in calcium and see if your craving dissipates. Calcium-rich foods include tofu or leafy green vegetables like kale, spinach, or arugula. Some forms of cheese contain good amounts of calcium and do not include additives and preservatives. Examples of these include mozzarella and feta cheese.

- Fatty Foods

If you find yourself craving fatty, carbohydrate-dense foods like muffins or high-fat baked goods, you could have an omega-3 deficiency. Omega-3 is a type of fatty acid, which is usually found in oils or fats. These specific types of fatty acids are called "essential fatty acids" because the interesting thing about omega 3, is that our bodies actually cannot produce it. This is what makes it essential, which means that we must ingest it for our bodies to have any at all. Because of this, you might see many people take Omega-3 supplements, or you may find eggs sold in the grocery store that have omega-3 written on the packaging.

So, if this is the case, what foods should you be eating to get this essential nutrient? Omega-3 can be found in the following food sources:

- Fish such as salmon and tuna

- Nuts and seeds like walnuts, flax seeds, or chia seeds- the types of seeds that you would add to smoothies or smoothie bowls.

Adding the foods listed above into your diet can help you to get this essential nutrient. By learning more about common cravings and what they could be telling you, you can begin to learn more about your body. This will help you to listen and observe what it is telling you, so that you are not restricting your diet and, in turn, keeping your body deprived of something it needs.

Chapter 2: Re-Framing Your Mind

In this chapter, we will examine intuitive eating rules #4 and #5 and look at how these ideas will come into play in your new lifestyle. These rules are critical in outling how you should think when adopting the intuitive eating lifestyle.

Intuitive Eating Rule #4: Recognize When You Are Full

It can be hard to determine how much you should eat or when you have had enough without eating to the point of feeling stuffed.

Many times, we keep eating until we are full, sometimes to the point of making ourselves feel physically ill. We want to avoid this, as the goal anytime you eat is to give your body what it needs so that it can function optimally for you. In this section, you are going to learn how to take care of your body, because stuffing it to complete fullness is not what it is asking for.

There are a few different ways that you can deal with this. Using these techniques, you can help yourself realize when you are satiated. Keep in mind, it will take some time to train your mind to understand when you have eaten enough. With enough practice, you will be able to recognize the signs of satiety much earlier. Below are a few ways you can begin recognizing when you are full.

1. Pay close attention to your body as you are eating. When you feel like you may be satiated, stop eating and wait for about twenty minutes. You will likely feel full then, but if not, you can always eat a bit more after the 20 minutes passes.

2. Before you eat, drink a glass of water. This will help you to eat just the right amount and not too much, as this will allow you to have something in your stomach already when

you begin eating. This will also help with your digestion as the water will allow everything to move smoothly along your digestive tract.

3. Another way to recognize when you are full is by eating more slowly. When we eat, it takes about twenty minutes for the hormone in our bodies that tells us that we are full to reach our brain. Our stomach signals to our brain that we are hungry, and that signal takes about twenty minutes to actually reach the brain. Thus, we want to make sure that we eat slowly so that we can precisely tell when we are full. If we eat very quickly, by the time we get the signal that we are full, we will have already eaten much more than we may have needed.

Intuitive Eating Rule #5: Eliminate Dietary Thinking

This rule will help you turn your mind away from dietary thinking and towards a newer, more productive way of viewing your relationship with food and hunger.

If you force yourself to change like a drill sergeant in an aggressive manner, you will end up being unnecessarily tough on yourself every day. The result will be feelings of failure and defeat.

Forcing yourself to do anything in life will not lead to long-lasting change. You will eventually become fed up with all of the rules you have placed on yourself, and you will be inclined to abandon the goal altogether.

If you approach change with rigidity, you will not allow yourself time or space to look back on your achievements and congratulate yourself. Thus, you may fall off of your plan into an even more extreme and unhealthy lifestyle than you had before. You may end up having a week-long binge and falling into worse habits of eating. To further illustrate this concept, I have outlined something called *The Deprivation Trap* below.

The Deprivation Trap is something that can occur when you approach dieting with a strict mindset. What this means is that you become stuck in something called a *thinking trap*. When this occurs, you become focused on what you can't have and what you are restricting yourself of, instead of what you *can* have. You become hyper-focused on everything you aren't allowing yourself to have. You then become resentful of the fact that you aren't able to just eat whatever you want.

After a while, because you are focusing so intently on what you can't have and the fact that you can't have it, you decide that you are just going to have it anyway. This decision comes from a feeling of anger and entitlement. The next thing you know, you have gone on a binge, and after restricting yourself completely for some time, you have now undone any progress you made in a single sitting.

You will then begin to feel terrible about yourself and what you have done, and will feel the need to punish yourself. Thus begins the cycle of deprivation.

It is quite difficult to avoid this trap when you are trying to make lifestyle changes through food deprivation. It is quite rare that a person, no matter how strong their willpower, will be able to completely deprive themselves of something without first easing themselves off of it. A sudden and strict deprivation is not natural to our brains and will leave us feeling confused and frustrated.

Instead of approaching your diet and eating habits with this kind of dietary thinking, intuitive eating encourages you to instead listen to what your body is telling you. By using your body as the guide for your personal eating schedule and plan, you will not fall into the deprivation trap.

Instead of following a diet plan that another person made for you, you will make your own rules. Nobody else knows your body as well as you do, so why let them tell you what you should and should not eat? Instead, listen from the inside, and that will be the only guide you need when it comes to eating.

Chapter 3: The Pitfalls of Emotional Hunger

This chapter contains a wealth of information about emotional hunger and emotional eating, as well as many strategies and tips for how you can conquer it. We will discuss the Intuitive Eating Rule #6 and define the term *Emotional Eating* for you to help you to understand it.

Also in this chapter, you will find information about emotional eating and how it affects your brain and your body. We'll cover some reasons why people emotionally eat and how to tell the difference between actual hunger and emotional hunger.

What Is Emotional Hunger?

First, let us begin by defining the term *emotional hunger*. This section will help you to determine whether this is something you suffer from.

Emotional hunger or emotional eating occurs when a person is suffering from emotional deficiencies of some sort. This includes lack of affection, lack of connection, or other factors like stress, depression, anxiety and general feelings of sadness or anger.

Therefore, to reduce the negative feelings they are experiencing or to feel better about them, they will find comfort through ingesting food. This is called emotional eating.

Some people turn to this type of eating on occasion, such as during a breakup or after a bad fight with someone. When this occurs several times in a week for a prolonged period, this type of eating can negatively impact a person's life. Over time, it can become a never-ending cycle of hopelessness that leads to bigger problems.

Real Hunger Versus Emotional Hunger

Sometimes it can be hard to tell when we are really hungry, and when we may be feeling as though food will make us feel better emotionally.

Real hunger is when our body needs nutrients or energy and is letting us know that we should replenish our it soon. This happens when it has been a few hours since our last meal, like when we wake up in the morning, or after a lot of strenuous activity such as a long hike. Our body uses hunger as a signal that it requires energy and that if it doesn't get it soon, it will begin to use stored energy sources as fuel. While there is nothing wrong with the body using its stored fuel, this signal is a sign that we should eat to replenish those energy stores.

Perceived hunger or emotional hunger is when a person thinks they are hungry, but their body doesn't require any more energy. This could happen for several reasons:

1. The brain notices that it is the time of day when you would normally eat, even if we have just eaten a short time before.
2. You are feeling stressed or anxious, and your body isn't sure of how to soothe this so it thinks that food may help.
3. When your emotional state makes you crave comfort and positive feelings, knowing that you can obtain these from certain foods.

Intuitive Eating Rule #6. Don't Eat Out Of "Emotional Hunger."

Emotional hunger occurs because eating foods that we enjoy makes us feel rewarded on a biological and chemical level within the brain. If you are wondering why a person would continue to eat emotionally when this is known to cause problems in their life, it is because the sense of reward that they feel encourages them to eat more. This intense feeling outweighs the possibility of future negative consequences as a result of eating too much.

How To Determine Whether Your Hunger Is Emotional Hunger Or Actual Hunger

In this section, we will look at the different types of hunger and how you can tell them apart. This will help you to distinguish when you are hungry and when you may be turning to food to soothe your emotional state.

When we feel hungry, there are several questions we can ask ourselves to determine which category we fall into. Below, I have listed the questions to ask and what they can tell us about our hunger.

1. *When did I last have a meal?*

You should ask yourself this question because if you had a full meal less than 2 or 3 hours ago, it is likely that you are not experiencing actual hunger. Still, the hunger is coming from something else like an emotional need or boredom.

2. *How hungry am I?*

Go within and ask yourself how hungry you are. While you don't want to wait until you are starving and light-headed to eat, you want to be hungry enough to warrant eating. If you are not quite at a level where you could eat a meal, you probably aren't hungry enough to eat just yet.

3. *Am I still hungry now?*

If you feel hungry, try drinking a glass of water. Wait twenty minutes and see if you are still hungry afterward. If you are not, you could have just been hungry because of your emotional state.

4. Was there a change in my emotional state previously?

Sometimes, we will feel the need or the compulsion to eat right after we get some bad news or have an upsetting thought or conversation. Ask yourself if you felt the feeling of hunger directly after one of these occurrences or something that you know to be a trigger for your emotional hunger. If something like this has just happened, you may not have connected them as being related. By taking a minute to recognize this, you can decide that you may not actually be hungry and address the emotional issue instead.

5. Do I feel hungry again right after eating?

If we begin to eat or have a snack when we feel emotional hunger, you may feel good right afterward, but shortly after, it will not be resolved. This is another way to find out whether you are actually hungry or not. If you do decide to eat something and shortly after feel hungry again, you were likely not hungry for food but had an emotional need instead. Since this emotional need could not be resolved with food, you feel hungry and crave that positive feeling you get right after eating.

6. Do I feel guilty about eating?

If you eat when you are hungry, you will feel satisfied and ready to continue with your day. You will not feel any sense of guilt or shame about it because you were simply fueling your body. However, if you ate when you had a craving and you felt hunger, but it was an emotional need telling you that you were hungry, you may feel guilty or ashamed afterward about having eaten.

This feeling can indicate that you were not hungry but that you were trying to fill a void that was not filled by eating food.

The reason that hunger doesn't become improved or disappear after eating is that the body craves food for that positive feeling that we get after we eat. Eating certain foods or craving the addictive chemicals within the food, makes us feel rewarded and happy temporarily because of the reaction in our brain that is similar to taking a drug. Our mind enjoys this feeling, and it helps to lift our mood or take our mind off of our emotional turmoil for the moment.

The problem is that when these rewarding and positive feelings are gone, we return to feeling the way we did beforehand. The only way to truly resolve our emotions or feel better about something is to face them head-on. Trying to solve them by other means like eating or distracting ourselves will only work in the short term and will leave us feeling those same negative emotions after the distraction is gone.

In the next section, we are going to look at how you can begin to deal with your emotions in healthy and productive ways, without using food as a means of coping.

How Food Cravings Often Indicate Emotional Deficiencies

To assist you in your practice of dealing with your emotions safely, I will share some of the most common emotional deficiencies that people face. These emotional deficienies are the causes that lead people to seek out food as a means of coping. First, though, we will look at one of the most prominent theories behind this and how the study of emotional hunger is helping people who suffer from it to make beneficial changes in their lives.

While other types of cravings can occur (such as the cravings that pregnant women experience, or those that indicate nutrient deficiencies), there are some strategies that you can use to determine whether your cravings are being caused by a true emotional deficiency. This begins by examining which exactly foods you crave and when they crave them.

For example, if you feel like eating a pizza every time you experience high levels of stress, or if you are depressed and you begin eating a lot of chocolate, this could indicate emotional eating.

Conversely, if you crave fruits like a slice of watermelon on a hot day, you are likely just dehydrated, and your body is trying to get water from a water-filled fruit that it knows will make it more hydrated. This is an example of a regular craving that indicates your body is simply seeking water in the form of fruit. On the other hand, if you often feel hungry when you are at home, and you live in a house full of turmoil and frustration, this could indicate emotional hunger.

Examining things and situations like this leads scientists and psychiatrists to explore this concept in more depth and determine what types of emotional deficiencies can manifest themselves through food cravings.

Examples Of Emotional Deficiencies

There are several types of emotional deficiencies that can be indicated by hunger. We will explore these in more detail, in hopes that you will recognize some of the reasons why you may be experiencing disordered eating.

- Childhood Causes

If you think back on your childhood, think about how your relationship with food began. Maybe you were taught that when you behaved, you received food as a reward. Maybe when you were feeling down, you were given food to cheer you up. Maybe you turned to food when you were experiencing something negative. Any of these experiences could lead someone to suffer from emotional eating in adulthood. This tumultuous relationship with food was something you may have learned early on.

This type of disordered eating is quite difficult to break as it has likely been a habit for many years. When we are children, we learn habits without knowing, and we often carry these habits into our adult lives. While this is no fault of yours, recognizing it as a potential issue is important to make changes.

- Covering Up Emotions

Another emotional deficiency that can manifest itself in emotional eating and food cravings is the effort to cover up our feelings. Sometimes we would rather distract ourselves and blanket our emotions than to face them head-on.

In this case, our brain may make us feel hungry to distract us from the emotions we are experiencing. When we have a quiet minute where these feelings or thoughts would pop into our minds, we can cover them up by deciding to prepare food and eat. We convince ourselves that we are "too busy" to acknowledge our feelings because we have to deal with our hunger.

The fact that it is hunger that arises in this scenario makes it very difficult to ignore and very easy to deem as a necessary distraction since, after all, we do need to eat to survive. This can become a problem, however, if your body does not require nourishment.

If there is an issue in your life that you think you may be avoiding or if you tend to be very uncomfortable with feelings of unrest, you may be experiencing this type of emotional eating.

- Feeling Empty Or Bored

When we feel bored, we often decide to eat or convince ourselves that we are hungry. This occupies both our mind and our time, while making us feel less bored, sometimes to the point of feeling positive or happy.

We can also eat when we are feeling emotionally empty. This void can be a general feeling of dissatisfaction with life, or the feeling of lacking something important.

When we feel this way, the food will quite literally be ingested to fill the void. This will inevitably lead to an unhealthy cycle of trying to administer our emotions with something that will never actually work. We will become disappointed every time and continue trying to fill this void with material things like food or shopping.

Examining the true reason behind the void is difficult, but will help you greatly in the long term. Being able to recognize when hunger is masking another issue is key to ending disordered eating for good. Doing so will also help you to identify ways to fill the emotional void that can be more healthy and productive, such as group fitness or taking up a new hobby.

- Affection Deficiency

Another emotional deficiency that could manifest itself as food cravings is an affection deficiency. This type of deficiency can be feelings of loneliness, feelings of a lack of love, or feelings of being undesired. If a person has recently gone through a breakup, or if a person has not experienced physical intimacy in quite some time, they may be experiencing an affection deficiency.

This type of emotional deficiency will often manifest itself in food cravings as we will try to gain feelings of comfort and positivity from the good tasting, drug-like foods that have allure us.

- Low Self-Esteem

Another emotional deficiency that may be indicated by food cravings is a low level of self-esteem. Low self-esteem can cause people to feel down, unlovable, inadequate, and overall negative and sad. This can make a person feel like eating enjoyable foods will make them feel better, even if only for a few moments.

Low self-esteem is an emotional deficiency that is difficult to deal with, as it affects every area of a person's life. This includes their love life, social life and career. Sometimes, people have reported feeling like food was always there for them when nobody else was. While this is true, they will often be left feeling more empty and down on themselves after giving into cravings.

- Mood

A general low mood can cause emotional eating. While we all have general low moods or bad days, if this makes you crave food multiple times per week, this could become emotional eating.

- Depression

Suffering from depression also can lead to emotional eating. Depression is having a continuous low mood for months on end which can cause a person to turn to food for comfort and a lift in spirits. This, in turn, becomes emotional eating.

- Anxiety

Having anxiety can lead to emotional eating, as well. Both general anxiety (constant levels of anxiety) and situational anxiety (triggered by a situation or scenario) can lead to emotional eating.

You have likely heard of the term *comfort food* to describe certain foods and dishes. The reason for this is because they are usually foods that are rich in carbohydrates, fats, and are generally heavy. These foods bring people a sense of comfort and are often turned to by people suffering from anxiety, because they help to provide temporary relief. These foods make them feel calmer and more at ease. However, this only lasts for a short time and their anxiety usually gears up again.

- Stress

Stress eating is probably the most common form of emotional eating. While constantly being on the go, stress is increasingly more common in today's world. While this does not become an issue for everyone experiencing stress, it is a problem for those who consistently turn to food to ease their stress. Some people are always overwhelmed, and they will constantly be looking for ways to ease this feeling.

Food is one of the ways that people make themselves feel better and take their minds off of their stress. As with all of the other examples we have seen above, this is not a lasting resolution, and it becomes a cycle. Similar to the cycle of emotional eating that we discussed, the same can be said for stress. Unlike emotional eating, stress eating can make you feel more tense, as you feel like you have done something you shouldn't have, which causes you to become more frazzled. Thus, the cycle ensues.

There are many different emotional causes for the cravings we experience. A person's emotional eating experience is unique and personal to them.

You may find that you experience a combination of the emotional deficiencies just mentioned. Many of these can overlap, such as anxiety and depression, which are often seen together in a single person. Whatever your struggles are, know that there is hope for recovery. This is what the rest of this book is designed to help you with, as it will allow you to reframe your relationship with food.

How To Deal With Your Emotions Without Relying On Food

As you can see from what we have discussed so far, recognizing the struggles you face involving food will help you to recover from being a person who uses food as a coping mechanism. This will help you to move towards being a person who has a healthy relationship with eating and become someone who can deal with their emotions in healthier ways.

Recognizing the things with which you struggle will help you to figure out how to deal with them. Nobody can force anybody else to make a change, especially an entire lifestyle change. So, recognizing the struggles that you are facing will allow you to be in charge of your journey to recovery.

Recognizing the food-related struggles you face will also help you to have a better relationship with your body. Instead of viewing your body as something that you dislike, you can begin to love it and care for it. You can do this by providing it with nourishment, clean energy, and adequate hydration. Viewing your body as something to care for as it carries you around all day will allow you to shift your view of yourself and see your body in a more positive light. You will begin to view it as something that you work together with instead of something that you work against.

Recognizing your struggles will also help you to have a better relationship with your mind. Understanding how your mind works will help you to better take care of it. You will be able to recognize your feelings and what they could be caused by, and then treat them in a way that will help it to feel better.

Bettering your relationship with food and your relationship with your body will also improve your relationship with your mind. This is because you will begin to provide it with what it needs. Which will, in turn, lead to better cognitive functioning, control over impulses and decision-making.

Doing some serious and deep self-reflection is not an easy process but a necessary one when it comes to healing yourself and changing your ingrained habits. Looking deep within and asking yourself the right questions will help you to take the first step.

The first step is to acknowledge your issues and find the sources of them. Finding the sources will tell you exactly what you need to face and deal with to find lasting change in the form of this new intuitive eating lifestyle.

If changing your life is done as a distraction from the underlying issues, the change will not be lasting. These issues will rise to the surface again eventually, and they will manifest themselves in strong cravings. I want you to be able to change your life permanently, and to do this we will begin with some deep self-reflection. This step is the most crucial and perhaps the most difficult. Try to keep your mind focused on the life you want because it can be yours. You deserve happiness and health! You will get out of this workbook what you put in, so take your time as you go through this chapter and try to get in touch with the deeper parts of yourself.

We will begin the self-reflection with some questions that you can ask yourself to get into a self-examination mindset. Complete this workbook, and you will be well on your way to dealing with your emotions.

The first question you will ask yourself is a rather obvious one, but this will make it easy for you to get a start on your self-examination.

1. Do I feel like I struggle with emotional eating?
Yes _____ No _____

2. Do I wish to find out the underlying causes of my emotional eating?
Yes _____ No _____

3. Do I feel like it is time for a lifestyle change in terms of my eating habits?
Yes _____ No _____

4. Have I been diagnosed with any mood-related disorders (such as depression, bipolar disorder, or anxiety)?
Yes ____ No____

If your answer is yes, you skip the next set of questions. If you answered No, or you are unsure, answer the following:

5. Do I have long periods of low mood or an anxious state?
Yes ____ No ____

6. Have I been feeling this way for the last 3 to 6 months?
Yes ____ No ____

7. Do I often feel disconnected from my life?
Yes ____ No ____

8. Do I often feel nervous and worried about worst-case scenarios?
Yes ____ No ____

9. Do I often catastrophize in my head when thinking about things that are to come?
Yes ____ No ____

10. Do I often feel drastic swings between very high moods (like happy, excited and motivated) and very low moods (sad, down, hopeless)
Yes ____ No ____

If you answered mostly Yes to the 6 questions above, you might suffer from a mood-related disorder. While this questionnaire is not conclusive and is not sanctioned by a doctor or a medical professional, this could give you a bit of direction when it comes to your mood, your emotions, and the causes of your emotional eating. I encourage you to dig deeper if you feel like a question resonates with you. Positive change will come out of finding and addressing the root of your problem.

Knowing that the cause could be something like depression, anxiety, or other mood disorders can help to give you some clarity about your mental state. If you think this could be the case, consider visiting your doctor (or someone knowledgable in these areas) to talk about this further.

How To Feel Your Emotions

It is very important to notice and address your feelings, as they can have many important things to tell you.

Pay attention to your thoughts. Whenever you feel a negative emotion, work backwards. Try to figure out what thoughts were just on your mind before you felt negative emotions. Emotions that you should be looking out for are stress, anxiety, self-loathing, sadness, demotivation, anger, and frustration. These emotions are the ones that typically cause a person to choose instant gratification.

Just like how you will be paying attention to the thoughts that occurred before feeling a negative emotion, pay attention to the thoughts that occurred before feeling a positive one. Typically, when a person is feeling positive emotions, it creates more motivation and inspiration to reach goals.

One great way to begin feeling through your emotions is by self-reflecting on them and noticing when they are causing your struggles with food. Recognizing your triggers is important because this will help you to understand the differences between feeling emotional hunger and feeling actual hunger.

What are some triggers related to your emotions or specific emotions that make you seek comfort in the form of food? Are there any triggers that you experience that cause your emotional deficiencies to flare up? For example, you may think the following:

- "When I feel scared, I begin to crave sweets."
- "When I am lonely, I want a cookie."
- "When I get stressed, I want a salty snack."

If you become hungry, you can look back on your day or the last hour and determine if any of your triggers were present. If they were, then you will be able to determine that you are likely experiencing emotional hunger, and you can take the appropriate steps instead of giving in to the cravings blindly.

When you experience a trigger that causes one of your emotional deficiencies to come to the surface, this will be a time that you will most likely to turn to food as a means of comfort and as a way to self-soothe. Recognizing what these triggers are will help you to recognize when to intervene in your thought process.

Instead of giving into cravings after an emotion triggers your feelings of loneliness, you will intervene and say to yourself, "A trigger just occurred, so I am going to call a friend and talk instead of eating what I crave."

Intuitive Eating Rule #7. Listen to Your Body

The seventh intuitive eating rule is one that is very important when it comes to intuitive eating, and it is arguably the most important of them all.

Intuitive eating comes down to listening to your body, so this list would not be complete without rule #7. While it may seem obvious to some, to many other people, listening to your body is quite a difficult thing to do. In a society where there are so many distractions, something seemingly as simple as listening to your inner self can be quite a difficult task. In this section, we are going to look at some tips for listening to your body and how this will benefit you when it comes to emotional eating.

How To Eat When You Are Hungry

When we discussed emotional eating in the previous section of this chapter, we looked at a list of questions that you can ask yourself when determining whether you are genuinely hungry or if you are experiencing emotional hunger.

If you ask yourself all of the above questions, and you determine that you are experiencing actual hunger, the next step is to take action and nourish your body with healthy and delicious foods.

While some people determine that they are experiencing actual hunger, a problem arises though when they subsequently begin to feel a series of self-judgments and second guesses. These can be thoughts like the following:

- Should I eat?
- Do I deserve to eat?
- Am I going to eat or am I going to wait?

When you live according to the intuitive eating mindset, you are not going to enter this spiral of thoughts, but you will instead feed your body.

The key to intuitive eating is to eat when you are hungry, but not when you are ravenous. If you are only mildly hungry, you can likely stand to wait a little bit to eat. As a rule of thumb, when you start to become mildly hungry, begin to prepare your meal so that by the time you finish, you are at the perfect level of hunger as you sit down to eat. If we wait to eat until we are ravenous, we will have let our blood sugar drop to quite a low level and we will likely have begun to get light-headed, irritable, and have difficulty with decision making. If you feel like this when you are beginning to eat, you will want to make a note to eat a bit earlier next time.

How To Begin Listening To Your Body

If you are experiencing a flurry of negative emotions when you decide that it is time to eat, you will be focused on your emotional state rather than on tasting and enjoying the food that you are eating.

While we have touched on this briefly in the book already, the reason that emotional hunger can become such a problem for so many people is that your body learns over time that eating certain foods (such as those containing processed sugars or salts like fast food and quick pastries), makes it feel rewarded even though the end result is often guilt.

When you are sad or worried, your body feels negative and looks for ways to remedy this. Your brain then decides that eating those fast foods will make its emotional state more positive. As a result of this process, (which happens entirely in the background of your mind), you will consciously feel a craving for those foods. These foods usually include sugary snacks or salty fast-food meals, and you may not even be aware of why you crave them.

If you decide to give in to this craving and eat something like a microwave pizza snack, your body will feel rewarded and happy for a brief period, which reinforces to your brain that craving food to make itself feel better has worked. If you end up feeling down and guilty that you ate something that was unhealthy, your brain will again try to remedy these negative emotions by craving food, and a cycle of emotional eating will begin.

Emotional hunger and listening to your body go hand in hand, which is why they have been included in the same chapter of this book. By understanding your emotions and what they mean, you will make room to listen to your body without having to find an unhealthy way to distract yourself from uncomfortable feelings.

Listening to your body includes both mental and physical signs that your body is sending to you. We have already talked about emotional or mental signs, so now we are going to talk about the physical signs.

One of the best ways to begin listening to your body is by doing meditation, or by being mindful. We are going to talk about something called *mindful eating* later on in the book, but for now, we are going to focus on using mindfulness as a means of getting in touch with your physical body.

The Body Scan Practice is a technique that can be performed multiple times a day to help you identify what you are feeling physically and mentally. Using this technique, you can learn to release the stress carried in your body and mind. Most of the time, when you are stressed, it's very common for it to be held in different areas of your body in the form of tense shoulders, stomach pains, or side aches. A lot of the time, you likely aren't even aware of the stress that you are carrying in your body. During periods of extra stress, you may be feeling a lot of physical discomfort but not necessarily connect it with your emotions.

The body scan meditation method is effective in relieving stress not only from the mental aspect but in the physical aspect, as well. Research points to the fact that there are numerous physical and psychological benefits to relieving tension and relaxing your body. Relieving physical tension has been proven to lower psychological stress even when you aren't using any external stress relief efforts for the mind. Relieving tension in your body can decrease overall lower levels of stress, which then leads to less physical tension. This meditation works to break the vicious cycle of mental and physical tension that feed off each other. Due to this, the body scan meditation is a very effective and useful meditation technique that allows you to remain both physically and mentally relaxed. ("Body

Scan Meditation", 2019). It can help you return to a calm state when you notice that you've become too tense. Here is how to perform body scan meditation.

1. Find a comfortable place where you can sit down and fully relax your body. It's easier if you are lying down, but sitting down is effective as well. Try to find a position that is comfortable for you but not so comfortable that you may fall asleep easily. Bring awareness to your breath. Let it slow down and start breathing from deep within your belly instead of your chest. Let your abdomen expand and then contract with each breath you take. If you find your shoulders moving up and down while breathing, bring your attention to your belly and allow the breathing from there. Pretend as if it's a balloon inflating and deflating your abdomen as you take each breath.

2. This is where we begin to do the actual 'body scan.' Pretend that there is a scanner above you (if you are lying down) or in front of you (if you are sitting down). Imagine that this scanner expels a laser beam that is slowly scanning your body. It begins at the top of your head. Bring your awareness to where that scanner is and slowly move it down your body. Do you notice any tension that you feel as you move the scanner through your body? Do you feel any tightness on your shoulders, neck, back, or stomach? Do you feel any sensations of pain, whether it's subtle or sharp? Are you feeling any areas of concentrated energy in your body? If you notice and feel something that is off, try to acknowledge it and think about why it might be. If there is tension, release it and move on. Continue to scan your body all the way from your scalp to your ears, cheeks, chin and neck. This becomes more automatic and much easier with

practice to the point that you will be able to do this very quickly and with less effort.

3. Make sure you're bringing attention to areas that you've discovered that have uncomfortable sensations. Breathe into them and watch what happens. Try to imagine the tension leaving your body through the exhale of your breath. A lot of people notice that the tight feeling becomes more intense at first, but continuing to meditate through the discomfort allows it to dissipate. Keep your awareness focused on that feeling for a few moments; make sure you are staying present. Feel free to give yourself a light massage in that area if it helps and move on to the next part of your body when you're ready.

4. Continue to do this scan with each area of your body, moving from your head to your toes. Make a note of how you feel and which body parts are holding stress. Helping release tension in your body now will allow you to be more aware of it in the future so you can relieve it as you feel those sensations.

Try to practice the body scan meditation several times throughout the day or during times where you feel stressed. If you are short on time, you can do an abbreviated version of this meditation by sitting down and bringing awareness to any place in your body where you feel tension.

Chapter 4: Making Peace With Your Body

In this chapter, we are going to learn about the importance of making peace with your body and how you can begin to do this. We are first going to look at the eighth rule of intuitive eating and how this relates to coming to terms with your body.

Intuitive Eating Rule #8. Don't Self Judge

This rule is very difficult for many people.

You cannot fully embrace the practice of intuitive eating if you have nagging feelings of self-judgment each time you take a bite of food or decide that you are going to eat lunch when you are hungry. In this section, we are going to look at some strategies for dealing with and overcoming self-judgment.

Let us examine this intuitive eating rule with an example. Let's say you are trying to focus on healthy eating, and you find that you have had trouble doing so. Maybe you ate a cupcake, or maybe you had a soda at breakfast. From the perspective of a traditional diet mentality, this would pose a problem for the diet, and this can lead to feelings of regret and disgust. You would likely be beating yourself up and feeling terrible about the choice you have made.

It is very important to avoid beating yourself up or self-judging for falling off the wagon. This may happen sometimes. What we need to do is focus not on the fact that it has happened, but on how you are going to deal with it and react to it.

There are a variety of reactions that a person may have to this type of situation. We will now examine the five most common reactions and their characteristics.

1. The person may feel as though their progress is ruined and that they might as well begin another time again, so they go back to their old ways and may not try again for some time. This could happen many times over as they will fall off each time and then decide that they might as well give up this time and try again, but each time it ends the same.

2. The person could fall off of their diet plan and tell themselves that this day is a write-off and that they will begin the next day again. The problem with this method is that continuing the rest of the day as you would have before you decided to make a change will make it so that the next day is like beginning all over again, and it will be very hard to begin again. They may be able to begin the next day again, and it could be fine, but they must be able to heavily motivate themselves if they are to do this. Knowing that you have fallen off before makes it so that you may feel down on yourself and feel as though you can't do it, so beginning again the next day is very important.

3. Similar to the previous case, the person may fall off, but instead of deciding that the day is a write-off, they tell themselves that the entire week is a write-off, and they then decide that they will pick it up again the next week. This will be even harder than starting the next day again. Multiple days of eating whatever you like will make it very hard to go back to making the healthy choices again afterward.

4. After eating something that they wish they hadn't, that wasn't a healthy choice, they will decide not to eat anything for the rest of the day. This is done to avoid eating too many calories or too much sugar. It may be the easy choice to decide that the next day they will begin again. This is very difficult on the body as you are going to be quite hungry when bedtime rolls around. Instead of forgiving yourself, you are punishing yourself, and it will make it very hard not to reach for chips late at night when you are starving and feeling down.

5. This reaction is the best for success and will make it much more likely that you will succeed long-term. If you fall off at lunch, let's say, because you are tired and in a rush, and you grab something from a fast-food restaurant instead of going home for lunch, there is a way to deal with it. First off, you will likely feel like you have failed and may feel quite down about having made an unhealthy choice. Instead of starving for the rest of the day or eating only lettuce for dinner, you will put this slip up at lunch behind you, and you will continue your day as if it never happened. You will eat a healthy dinner as you planned, and you will continue with the plan. You will not wait until tomorrow to begin again; you will continue as you would if you had made that healthy choice at lunch. The key to staying on track is being able to bounce back. The people who can bounce back mentally are the ones who will be most likely to succeed. Without question, you will need to maintain a positive mental state. This will help you to look forward to the rest of your day and the rest of your week in just the same way that you were before you had a slip-up. One bad meal out of the entire week is not going to ruin all of your progress and recovering from emotional eating is largely a mental game. It is more about mindset than anything else, so we must never underestimate the role that our thinking plays in our success or failure.

How To Make Peace With Your Body

Self-care is one of the best ways to begin making peace with your body. There are numerous ways that you can practice self-care, and they can be different for everyone. In this section, I will outline some ways that you can practice self-care to begin feeling more positive about yourself and your body and begin changing your internal environment.

- You Are Worthy

This is a great exercise to use to remind yourself of everything that you love and appreciate about yourself and your life. Take time to write down all of the things that you love about yourself and your life. This will remind you of all of the positivity surrounding you and will serve to uplift you.

- Limit Negative Influences

By limiting the negative influences in your life, you are making a statement to yourself. You are showing yourself that you place importance on preserving your mental health. When you remove negative influences and limit your exposure to things or people that make you feel negative, you are prioritizing yourself. This is a great way to practice self-care and can give you a sense of worth.

- Support System

Finding a positive and uplifting support system helps improve and preserve your mental health. This can be one person or a group of people. Your support system can include family, friends, or acquaintances, as long as they support you in your journey and help you to feel positive about yourself. Some examples of places that you can find a support system include Facebook groups, support groups, weight loss support groups and book support groups. Not only will a support system help you to move toward positivity, but when you begin to make changes in your life, your support system will help by supporting you in maintaining these changes.

- Journaling

Another exercise that you can do to change your mindset is to write down all of the limiting beliefs you think you possess. Next, try to write down where you believe they came from. For example, consider where you may have learned to think in this way. Having this information written down in front of you can help you to begin reforming your inner beliefs, as awareness is the first step to change.

How To Get Away From Self-Judgement

Self-judgement is something that everybody deals with to some degree. In this section, we are going to look at how you can take back the reins when it comes to your thoughts and feelings about yourself and how you can begin to shift them.

- Be aware

Awareness is the first step that needs to be taken to recognize your inner-critic and to reshape it into something less critical and more supportive. Try to pay attention the next time you are feeling distracted, tense, or anxious. Try to identify whose voice is the voice of your inner critic. Try to find the situation where this voice awakens. It allows yourself to dig deep and identify the most vulnerable feelings during situations where your inner critic is awake. These feelings or these situations are likely what your inner critic is trying to protect you from feeling. However, by protecting you, they are holding you back from meeting your full potential.

When people have developed unhelpful thinking processes, it is hard to make decisions to benefit their future self because their thoughts create negative emotions that drive away motivation. Some people argue that by simply increasing your willpower, thus overcoming the need for instant gratification, you will be able to fix your situation. This belief, however, is not an effective solution for long-lasting change. In this section, we are going to look at a variety of ways that you can begin to combat those limiting beliefs and the negative self-talk that goes on in your mind.

- Remind Yourself To Be Positive

As we learned, bad habits are built through many years, and no amount of willpower can handle overcoming that many bad habits in a person's life. Rewiring your brain to minimize the amount of negativity you feel in the first place is a much more efficient method to approach this problem.

- Catch Yourself Thinking According To Your Limiting Beliefs

Often, if the person had just paid attention to their thought process, they would be able to catch themselves before their mind automatically spiraled to a place of complete de-motivation. By catching yourself before you get there, you can prevent yourself from falling into your negative thought patterns that are limiting you and holding you back.

- Show Yourself Evidence Against Your Limiting Belief

Showing yourself evidence that supports or doesn't support the thoughts that are on your mind will help you to change your limiting beliefs. By showing yourself evidence, you can cancel out those negative thinking styles and give yourself the confidence and motivation to overcome any situation.

Often, people who are stuck in a mindset of, "I'm going to fail and embarrass myself anyway, so why bother?" will choose to not prepare. This leads to a feeling of failure when they inevitably do not achieve success. This further solidifies their limiting belief.

When your inner critic begins to tell you that you can't do a certain thing, or you're not good enough, or you're not worthy enough, simply find evidence within your past life experiences that challenge or discount this belief. Prove your inner critic wrong and show them why holding you back is only going to do more harm than if you failed whatever task you were planning to do. The more you tell your inner critic this, the more they will learn to listen to you and help you in another way that is not just preventing you from doing things.

- Ask For Support From Your Inner Critic

If your inner-critic is telling you that you are going to embarrass yourself, you can prove it wrong. You can do this by using evidence-based arguments and then asking for its support by saying "This is a difficult challenge for me, and I want to overcome it. I need you to support me, regardless of the outcome."

Remember, your inner critic is just another version of yourself. Be kind to it even if it's not being kind to you. Showing yourself, kindness is very important in our case.

- Negotiate With Your Limiting Beliefs To Change Them

When you notice these voices and statements that are going on in your brain which are related to your limiting beliefs, you can then simply acknowledge them and begin to negotiate with your inner critic. Let them know that you thank them for looking out for you, but you are confident in your ability to make decisions for yourself. You can let them know that even though you may fail and feel embarrassed, it is still better than a lifetime of holding yourself back. Since your inner critic is a part of you, it can listen to reason as long as you allow yourself to be reasoned with.

- Surround Yourself With Positive People

Surrounding yourself with people that can encourage you and foster positivity will also change your inner-critic's opinion. Often, hearing positive compliments from other people holds heavier weight in your mind when compared to you telling yourself the same thing. Try spending time with people who are supportive of your goals and the changes that you are looking to make in your life. It will make your journey a little bit easier.

Limiting beliefs and negative self-talk, as well as negative body-image, can lead a person to feel terrible about themselves, often to the point of feeling like they hate themselves. As I mentioned earlier, to make lasting changes, we are going to work on loving oneself instead of hating oneself. By seeing your body in a positive light, appreciating it for all of the things it allows you to do, you will begin to make choices with the health of your body in mind. This will lead to lasting, positive changes for your physical and mental health.

- Be Gentle with Yourself

It is important to be gentle with ourselves because we are usually our own toughest examiner. We look at ourselves very critically and we often think that nothing we do is good enough. We must be gentle with ourselves so as not to discourage ourselves. We must not put ourselves down, or make ourselves feel bad about what we are working so hard to accomplish. We must remind ourselves that everything in life is a process and does not happen instantly, and we mustn't tell ourselves to "hurry up and succeed," as we often do.

When you fall off track, you must not beat yourself up for this. It is important to be gentle with yourself. Beating yourself up will only cause you to turn into a spiral of negativity and continue to talk down to yourself. This will make you lose motivation and will make you feel like you are a failure. Having this state of mind will make it difficult not to turn to food for comfort.

You must avoid this entire process by avoiding beating yourself up in the first place. If you don't beat yourself up and instead encourage yourself, instead of thinking that it is too hard and then turning to food for comfort, you will not feel the need to find comfort at all. Instead, you will talk to yourself positively and encourage yourself from within. Then, instead of making yourself feel bad, you will instead make yourself feel motivated. You will be ready to continue on your journey.

Even if you don't fall off of the plan, it is still important to talk to yourself nicely and with encouragement. You must recognize that changing your behaviors that are ingrained in your life is no small feat. You must encourage yourself just like you would encourage someone else. Think of it as if you were talking to a good friend of a family member who was going through this instead of you. What would you say to them? How would you say it? You would likely be quite gentle and loving in your words. You would likely tell them that they were doing a great job and to keep it up. This is exactly how you want to speak to yourself from within and the exact types of words and phrases that you want to use. If we spoke to our friends the way we speak to ourselves most of the time, they would be quite hurt. Thus, we must remember this when trying to motivate ourselves, and we must be gentle.

Another way to be gentle with yourself is to avoid being too restrictive in the beginning. You must understand that it will be a challenge, and easing into this new lifestyle will be best. Beginning by making small changes and then adding more and more changes as you go will be a good way for your mind and body to get used to the changes. If you dump a lot of changes on yourself too quickly, this will feel like a burden for both your mind and body.

Chapter 5: Exercise Like Never Before

In this chapter, we are going to look at our final intuitive eating rule, and then we will spend some time discussing the importance of exercise and how it relates to intuitive eating.

Intuitive Eating Rule #9. Exercise Using Intuitive Movement

The ninth and final intuitive eating rule does not involve eating, but instead involves movement. Movement is an important part of overall health and wellbeing, which is why it is included in this list of rules. We will begin by looking at what intuitive movement is, and then I will share with you how you can begin making it a part of your life.

What Is Intuitive Movement?

Intuitive movement is the practice of moving according to the needs and wishes of your body. It can be viewed in the same way as intuitive eating, except with the movement of your body instead.

How Can Intuitive Movement Benefit You?

Exercise is great for our body, mind, and overall health. Adding an exercise regime into your life is as important, if not more, than any other measures you take to maintain your health. Exercise has been proven to help with a variety of things in life such as stress, impotence, and cellular repair. As you know, all of our body systems work together to form the person that we are. If one of them isn't functioning quite as well as it should be, all of the other systems feel it too. Exercise works on all of these systems at the same time, and if one of them isn't firing on all cylinders, exercise will help that system to wake up, improve, and stay healthy.

Exercising will show you what your body can do and how strong it is, which in turn will make you feel stronger mentally. Exercising will help you take your mind off of those nagging cravings and will give you more clarity overall. You are then able to look deep inside at those cravings and the emotional issues that are causing them. Exercise will help in all aspects of your life and will help you to continue reaching for recovery.

For any level of exercise, challenging your body in new ways will be beneficial in so many aspects of your life. In addition to its effects on the brain, body, and mood, it will help with your health in the long-run and the ease with which you will be able to complete everyday tasks like climbing the stairs or throwing a ball to your child. The goal is to make this a part of the new lifestyle you are working towards, which will make it so ingrained in your life that you will not want to be without it.

There are also chemical benefits to exercising that will assist both your body and mind. When we exercise, our brain releases chemicals that tell us we enjoy the effects that the exercise is giving us. This feeling is known as "runner's high," and it is that elation you feel after you run a long-distance or complete a workout.

When you are feeling sad, and you exercise, your mood will lift because of this runner's high. For this reason, it is not important what kind of physical exercise you do, but rather the fact that you simply engage in exercise period. Doing this regularly will help you feel motivated and will keep your mood positive.

This feeling of *runner's high* can be compared to the rewarded feelings that high-sugar foods give us. The difference is that with runner's high, the feelings of elation and accomplishment last way longer than the rewarded feelings we get from eating food.

Fast food makes our brains feel happy, but our body feels heavy and lethargic. Exercise, as I mentioned, makes your body feel great, and this is why the effects of runner's high are so long-lasting.

Similarities And Differences Between Intuitive Movement And Other Types Of Movement

Many people begin following some type of exercise plan to get in shape or to lose weight. Sometimes, this does not lead to success. People often end up having to try to force themselves to perform exercise that doesn't feel good for their body, that has not been personalized for them, and which they find no enjoyment in. This often lasts for a week or two, after which the person becomes fed up and decides that having to push themselves to perform the exercise plan is not worth the potential benefits.

On the other hand, intuitive movement involves a deeper motivation and an enjoyment factor that is not often present in other kinds of exercise regimes. If you enjoy the movement, you are much more likely to want to perform it, and you will not even need to force your body to do it, as you will genuinely want to take part in it.

As I mentioned earlier in this chapter, I am going to show you how all of the rules of intuitive eating can be applied to intuitive movement. Here, I will break down each one of them and show you how this kind of intuitive mindset can be applied to many different areas of your life to give you a new way of viewing yourself.

- *Intuitive Eating Rule #1. Adhere to Your Hunger*

This first rule is related to hunger and eating in particular, but if we instead change it to "Adhere to your body's wishes" in terms of movement, this can be understood to mean that we must listen to and follow our body's desires when it comes to movement and exercise.

- *Intuitive Eating Rule #2. Say No to The Diet Industry*

The diet industry often involves an exercise component that is rooted in the same basic principles as the diet plans that are trendy today. For example, if you are on a no carbohydrate diet, this often comes with the expectation that you will exercise in a certain way for a certain number of days in the week. By saying no to the diet industry, you are also saying no to boot camp-style exercise that you must force your body to do.

- *Intuitive Eating Rule #3. Don't Restrict What You Eat*

This intuitive movement principle is another important one. Don't restrict what you eat, and don't restrict how you move. For example, if you find joy in going for a long walk, don't restrict your movement by thinking that that is not an acceptable form of movement. When it comes to intuitive movement, anything goes, as long as it makes your body feel good!

- *Intuitive Eating Rule #4. Recognize When You Are Full*

Recognizing when you are full is important for intuitive eating, as well as recognizing when you are finished exercising. To avoid injury, pay attention to what your body is telling you and recognize when it has felt the benefits of your movement and when it is time to take a rest. Resting is an important part of intuitive movement.

- *Intuitive Eating Rule#5. Eliminate Dietary Thinking*

Eliminating dietary thinking, as well as eliminating the "boot camp" thinking when it comes to exercise, are both important. Instead of forcing yourself to attend a workout class that you hate or making yourself eat celery every day of the week, listen to your body and allow it to guide your movements.

- *Intuitive Eating Rule #6. Don't Eat Out of "Emotional Hunger."*

Emotional hunger is a concept that is quite specific to food, but it can also be applied to movement. If you are feeling negative emotions or if you are feeling down, you likely do not feel like moving your body at all, let alone partaking in some sort of exercise. When this happens, it is important to listen to your body and find out what will make it feel good in a healthy way. For example, you may wish to binge on a bag of chips in times of stress, but instead try to find something healthier to help you feel better. Exercise is a natural stress-reliever and anti-depressant. Maybe you wish to take a walk and get fresh air, or maybe you wish to leisurely swim in the pool. Whatever your body is telling you, follow that instead of trying to force yourself to do something that you will hate.

- *Intuitive Eating Rule #7. Listen to Your Body*

The number one principle of intuitive movement is to listen to your body. Your body knows what it wants and what it needs, so you must learn to trust this and listen to it. Over time you will get better at this, but for now, you will need to keep reminding yourself to do so, especially when it comes to exercise and movement.

- *Intuitive Eating Rule #8. Don't Self Judge*

Self-judging is something that everyone must deal with, and it can be quite a challenge to silence those voices in the back of your mind that are telling you all kinds of judgmental things. Instead of thinking, "I should be going to the gym right now," try to think positively about the movement that you have done or try to remember that your body needs rest, and if that is what it is asking for, then give it rest.

- *Intuitive Eating Rule #9. Exercise Using Intuitive Movement*

Exercising using intuitive movement is something that you will need to learn how to do, and it will likely involve a lot of unlearning as well. The first step is to learn to be gentle and kind with yourself and learn how to listen to your body and what it is telling you its needs are.

How To Begin Using Intuitive Movement

In this section, we are going to look at how you can begin using intuitive movement in your own life. Whether you are a seasoned runner or someone who has never exercised before in your life, there is an exercise routine out there for you that your body will enjoy. I will begin by sharing some different types of exercises that you can do. If you do not have much experience with exercise, you can begin to explore different types of movement to find out what your body enjoys the most.

Cardiovascular exercise and resistance training are two different types of exercise that people can benefit from. Cardiovascular exercise is the type of exercise that involves an elevated heart rate due to activities such as running, riding a bicycle, or swimming. This type of exercise is often referred to as "cardio." It is a type of exercise usually done for an extended period at a steady state.

Resistance training is a type of exercise that involves using weighs to build up your muscles by doing things like squats, push-ups, bicep curls, and so on. This is the type of exercise that you would often do if you go to a gym to exercise. Contrary to popular belief, this type of exercise will not make you bulky and muscular, especially if you are a woman. Instead, it will give you more tone and a leaner body.

When we engage in cardiovascular exercise, our heart rate increases, what this does is carry more oxygen to our muscles so that they can keep exercising. It also carries more oxygen to our brain. More oxygen and blood flow to the brain means that your brain will work more efficiently, more sharply, and with more clarity after you finish exercising. More blood flow to the brain also means that it will be generally healthier.

Exercising often and for a continuous period helps to keep the brain healthy and in working order. This helps with memory, decision making, and learning.

Exercise is also the most effective antidepressant. Many pills are prescribed to treat and beat depression, but the most effective and natural way of boosting your mood (and keeping it up) is through exercise.

When we exercise, we become stronger, faster, and more agile. This not only helps us to exercise better but it helps us in our everyday lives. Moving through life with more ease than before is a great feeling that can only be achieved through physical exertion. Our bodies are built to move, and they love it when we do! Our bodies are made to continually grow stronger the more we do, and this is what inevitably happens as soon as we begin exercising consistently. You will also begin to see aesthetic changes as well. You can see your muscles growing, your body toning, and your fat disappearing. These changes on the inside and the outside make us feel great about the body we live in, and about the progress we are making.

Taking the time to exercise and to stick with an exercise regime of any sort, as long as it makes your body and mind feel good, shows our body that we are willing to do the hard work that exercising takes, and it also shows our mind the same thing.

Do not be discouraged by your experience level when it comes to exercise, as everyone can benefit from it, and everyone must start somewhere. Below, I have given you several ideas for exercise, no matter the experience level you bring with you.

If you normally don't do much exercise or much walking around, begin by taking the stairs. Start by deciding to walk when you go to certain places, like to the store down the street or to a friend's house. Audiobooks and music can be a way of taking your mind off of what you are doing and make exercise more enjoyable. Beginning with this type of movement will get your body used to moving again and will get your muscles and joints working smoothly.

If you occasionally walk, like to the bus stop or the store on your lunch break, you can begin with a little bit more exercise than someone who is sedentary. Since your muscles and joints are likely somewhat used to being in a standing position, you can begin to jog a little bit. You can also jog after dinner around the block a few times, or jog to the store and walk back every few days. You could also take a yoga class if you wish or do some video-guided yoga at home.

On the other hand, you may already have a moderate level of walking included in your life and occasionally speed that up to a jog. If this is the case, you can begin to move your body around in new and different ways. Try doing some sit-ups and push-ups at home before or after your run. Alternatively, run to the neighborhood park and use the playground equipment to do some chin-ups, some jumps onto a step, or some running up and down the stairs. This will keep your heart rate up and teach your body new ways of moving while allowing your upper body muscles to get a bit of attention.

If you run frequently and you benefit from some bodyweight exercises now and again, try visiting a gym. At the gym, try doing some exercises with weights. You can try squatting, pressing some things overhead, and maybe some bicep curls. This will challenge your muscles in ways that your body weight cannot and take you to a new level of fitness and mood-boosting.

Finally, if you are an experienced runner, you are likely quite familiar with the feeling of runner's high. You are likely quite familiar with how exercise can change your mood around and take you from feeling hopeless to hopeful. If you want to try some new forms of exercise, try adding a gym routine using small weights. This will take your running to new heights and will give you a new type of exercise experience to break up the running days.

Continue to challenge yourself in new ways and teach your body new ways of moving. Exercise does nothing but good things, so keep up your routine.

There are some things to note if you are a woman. Since exercising helps women to regain some of the muscle mass lost with increasing age, it can be greatly beneficial for women to exercise into their older years. It is important to be aware of how to do this safely, though. It can be safer to stick to low-impact exercises, so avoid exercises that include jumping or any sort of quick, jarring movements. Instead, spending some time on an exercise bike (or a real bike) or an elliptical machine can be good as they both reduce impact and are therefore better for a woman's joints. Things like running involve more impact, so if you have joint pain, it is best to avoid this type of exercise. Further, lifting small weights or walking with weights in your hands can help you to build back some muscle. This will lead to an increase in your resting rate of metabolism. This is the number of calories your body burns when it is just sitting at rest to do things such as breathing or sitting. Your overall health will be greatly improved by an increase in muscle, the improvement of your joint health, and the lowered risk of diseases such as heart disease (which can be reduced by doing aerobic exercise).

If you are a person who hates running or traditional exercise, that is okay too! Luckily, there are numerous other exercises that do not fit into either of the two categories. These include exercises such as yoga, Pilates, high-intensity interval training and group training classes. While these are not considered to be traditional methods of exercise, they are no less valid than resistance training or cardiovascular exercise. Many people who are not too enthused about exercise wish to pursue methods that incorporate more of a social aspect or those that are slower in their movements. If this is what you prefer, this is just as valid as going for a run! There are even more ways to be active such as pursuing activities like gardening, dancing, hiking and kayaking. Any activity that raises your heart rate and brings you a sense of joy can be used as an exercise in combination with a diet change to provide you the health you are looking for.

Exercise meets you where you are, and your brain will gladly take any form of the new movement as a mood booster. When you enjoy the exercises that you are taking part in, you are much more likely to choose to engage in them more often and much less likely to find excuses to avoid them. By enjoying what you are doing, it will feel like a reward and not like a punishment. For this reason, be sure to choose a form of exercise that you enjoy.

The important thing here is that you are moving intuitively and that this is leading you to feel better in the body that you are in. Additionally, it should help you to realize that your body is an amazing vessel that allows you to do so many incredible and enjoyable things!

Chapter 6: Mindful Eating

In this chapter, we are going to look at mindfulness as it relates to eating. I will begin by defining mindfulness for you before moving onto something called mindful eating. This chapter will help you to learn how to be present in your life without distraction, which will lead to lifestyle improvement and a better relationship with food.

What Is Mindfulness?

Before we jump in, let's first learn about the basics of mindfulness. Mindfulness is most popularly achieved through the use of meditation. In modern society, psychology professionals describe meditation as a way to achieve mindfulness. It can be described as a method of focusing one's thoughts, and mind on an activity or object to train their awareness and attention. The goal of this is to help the person achieve clear-headedness and an emotionally calm, stable state. You may think that mindfulness sounds easy, but it is a very difficult activity to master.

Mindfulness is something that requires strong self-discipline. Simply just listening to a mindfulness podcast or going to one meditation class isn't going to help you become a mindful person.

How Can Mindfulness Benefit You?

The most popular reason that people decide to learn meditation is actually to achieve mindfulness to combat mental obstacles. If you are someone that lives a very fast-paced and stressful life, mindfulness and meditation can help you manage your thoughts and emotions to bring you more peace. Many doctors who specialize in the area of mental health have begun to study and even practice meditation and mindfulness techniques to promote a healthier brain and mind. Others take the practice of meditation and mindfulness to another level and aim to reach a high level of spirituality. When an individual can achieve mindfulness, they can increase their overall life satisfaction.

How To Begin Using Mindfulness In Your Life

You can practice mindfulness while washing the dishes, and nobody would know that you were 'meditating.' Mindfulness and meditation can come in many different forms, whether it's the act of meditating during a yoga session or if it's the act of simply being present in your life while folding the laundry. Mindfulness is a part of many different exercises and techniques to help people live a happier life.

There is, however, a basic form of mindfulness practice that you can use in any area of your life. We will look at some tips for how you can begin to practice this here, and you can then use this technique anytime you feel as though you are distracted or moving through your life on autopilot. You can even use it if you just need some time to be calm and in tune with your body and mind.

The most commonly practiced form of meditation is mindfulness meditation. This is also the most general type of meditation to help you facilitate mindfulness in all areas of your life. Mindfulness meditation is a type of mental training practice that involves you focusing your mind on your thoughts and sensations in the present moment (Agrawal, 2019). This includes your current emotions, physical sensations, and passing thoughts. Mindfulness meditation generally involves controlled breathing, mental imagery, self-awareness and muscle relaxation. It is typically easier for beginners to follow a guided meditation directing them throughout the whole process. It is extremely easy to drift away or fall asleep while in meditation if nobody is guiding you. Once you become more skilled in mindfulness meditation, you can do it without a vocal guide, but this requires strong mental capabilities.

Now, let's learn how you can practice mindfulness meditation. Most people do this for at least ten minutes each day. Even a couple minutes every single day can make a difference to your wellbeing. This is the basic technique that will help you get started:

1. Find a quiet place that you feel comfortable in—ideally, your home or someone where you feel safe. Sit in a chair or on the floor. Make sure your head and back are straight but are not tense.
2. Try to sort your thoughts and put aside those that are of the past and future. Stick to the thoughts about the present.
3. Bring your awareness to your breath. Make sure to focus on the feeling and sensation of air moving through your body as you inhale and exhale. Feel the way your belly rises and falls. Feel the air enter through your nostrils and leave through your mouth. Make sure to pay attention to the differences in each breath.
4. Watch every thought come and go. Act as if you are watching the clouds, letting them pass by you as you watch each one. Whether your thought is a worry, fear, anxiety, or hope - when these thoughts come up, don't ignore them or try to suppress them. Simply acknowledge them, remain calm, and anchor yourself with your breathing.
5. You may find yourself getting carried away in your thoughts. If this happens, observe where your mind went off to, and without making a judgment, simply return to your breathing. Keep in mind that this happens a lot with beginners; try not to be too hard on yourself when this happens. Always use your breathing as an anchor again.
6. As we near the end of the session, sit for a minute or two and become aware of where you physically are. Get up gradually.

You don't necessarily need to meditate to practice mindfulness. There are many other ways you can practice mindfulness without sitting down for a meditation session. However, I recommend you practice these methods when you are more experienced in mindfulness, as it will require much more focus and discipline.

Below are some examples of more specific scenarios in which you can practice mindfulness during your day. This will help you to reconnect with your inner self and with the environment around you.

- Doing the dishes

This is a great opportunity to practice meditation as typically nobody is trying to get your attention while you're doing the dishes. This perfect combination of alone time and physical activity makes a great window to try mindfulness.

Try to savor the feeling of the warm water on your hands. Savor the sensation and the appearance of the bubbles. Savor the smell of the dish soap, and the sound of pots and pans clunking under the water. If you're able to give yourself over to this experience, you'll end up with a refreshed mind and clean dishes!

- Brushing your teeth

Every single day you have to brush your teeth - this makes the normally boring task of dental hygiene a great opportunity to practice mindfulness.

Start by feeling your feet on the floor, the toothbrush in your hand, and the movement of your arm. Pay attention to this as you brush your teeth back and forth. A helpful tip is to pretend that there is a scanner - and that it is scanning your body from your feet up. Make sure to focus on the body part as the scanner moves from your feet to the top of your head.

- Driving

It is extremely easy for people to become mindless while driving. Especially if you're driving the same route day in and day out.

If you're driving to and from work, your mind typically wanders to what work tasks need to be completed that day, or the chores that you have to do once the day is over. Practice your mindfulness in the car as you're driving to keep yourself anchored inside the vehicle. Try to take in what's around you like the color of the car in front of you. The smell of the inside of your car. The way the steering wheel fits in your hands. Pay attention to all the noises you hear, from the music on the radio to the outside traffic noises. Whenever you find yourself wandering, bring your attention back to where you and your vehicle are in the moment.

- Exercising

Make your fitness routine an exercise in mindfulness by exercising away from screens and music. Focus on your breathing. Focus on where your feet are as you are moving. Sure, watching TV or listening to a podcast will make your run on the treadmill go by more quickly, but it won't do anything to quiet your mind. Allow yourself to feel the burn in your muscles and pay attention to how your body is reacting to the work out you are putting it through. Don't just ignore the pain of a muscle, acknowledge it, and let yourself feel the exercise.

- Bedtime

This is usually the time where you run around your home getting everything ready for your next long day, which is tomorrow. Don't battle too much with it; you know what needs to be done. Instead, stop trying to rush through it all and simply to try to enjoy the experience of doing the actual motions. Focus on the task at hand and don't think about the next task and the one after that. Leave yourself with enough time to not have to rush through the things you need to do. Again, any thoughts and anxieties that may come up this time, you may simply acknowledge them and let it pass.

- Mindful Eating

There are ways to eat which ensure that you are making the most of the time that you are eating, while also getting all of the nutrients that you need from your food. We will talk about something called mindful eating in more detail in the next section.

By paying attention to these important areas of your life and increasing your mindfulness in them, you can begin to see areas wherein which you can improve to help you live a happier life.

What Is Mindful Eating?

Mindful eating is when you really savor the moment, instead of being distracted by everything that is going on in your mind. Mindful eating is important as these are one of those tasks that we do numerous times per day. When we do a certain task repeatedly, our bodies will naturally try to automate that action to conserve energy.

However, when we eat mindlessly, we don't pay attention to the way food tastes, what we're eating, and how quickly we are consuming it. These bad automation habits are what causes us to mistreat our body. In this section, I will be teaching you the following:

- The basics of mindful eating
- How you can eat mindfully

- Exercises to help you practice this technique

The lack of mindful eating is something most of our population suffers from due to the increased pace of our lives. We typically find ourselves eating at work in front of our computer or eating dinner in front of the TV. Sometimes we may even eat during the commute to work! This seemingly small problem is actually one of the contributing factors in today's obesity and eating disorder problem. To combat this, we need to improve our ability to eat mindfully. Mindful eating uses the act of mindfulness to allow us to conquer common eating problems in our fast-paced lives (Beech, 2019).

The goal here is to shift focus from external thinking while eating, to joyfully delving into the eating experience itself. This is done to develop a new relationship with food. Here are a couple of points to help you identify when you are eating mindlessly.

- You are consistently eating until you are overly full or even feel sick
- You find yourself nibbling on food without really tasting it
- You aren't paying any attention to the foods you are eating and frequently eat in places that surround you with distractions
- You are rushing through your meals
- You have trouble remembering what you ate, or even the taste and smell of the last meal you've consumed

How Can Mindful Eating Benefit You?

- More Food Enjoyment in a Healthy Way

If you are feeling down emotionally when you do decide that it is time to eat, you may be focused on your emotional state and not really tasting or enjoying what you are eating. By practicing mindful eating, you will be present in your eating experience. This will help you to enjoy the taste of the food once again. It will also give you a chance to relax and relish in a few minutes of calm so that you can enjoy your food.

- Digestion

Ensuring that you eat mindfully comes with numerous benefits. One of these benefits is that it will help your body to digest more effectively. This will help you to get all the nutrients you need from your food.

- Decreases food cravings

Consciously eating will make you more aware of everything that you put into your mouth, and focusing on the experience of eating can help you to have fewer cravings and less desire to eat in between meals.

- Prevents overeating

This technique prevents overeating because you must pay attention to each bite that you put into your mouth. This will mean that you will be much more in tune with how full your body is.

- Improve your relationship with food

By using mindful eating, you will not be eating to make yourself feel better emotionally, but instead as nourishment for your precious body.

Practicing meditation is your first step in being able to achieve mindful eating. Allowing yourself to be mindful in your day to day life will bring new joys and satisfactions that have always been there but have not been noticed in some time, especially when it comes to a common activity like eating.

Steps Towards The Practice Of Mindful Eating

If you find yourself relating to the points I outlined in the first section; you may want to actively practice mindful eating. Follow these quick exercises below to begin increasing your level of mindfulness while eating.

- **Exercise #1: Prioritize your mealtimes.**

Try to isolate a 15-minute block to sit down and enjoy your meal. Don't eat on the go or skip meals because you're 'too busy.' Make sure you are always making time to eat at least three meals per day, no matter how busy you are.

- **Exercise #2: Avoid distractions while you are eating.**

It is impossible to enjoy eating your food when your attention is somewhere else. Try asking yourself how often you eat while in front of the TV, in the car, or in front of the computer. Eating under these circumstances is not mindful, and this can lead to overeating, choosing unhealthy options, or not enjoying the experience of your meal (Beech, 2019).

- **Exercise #3: Avoid being rushed around during meal times.**

Schedule a time block to eat your meal when you don't have any distractions around you. Even eating with a coworker or a friend may be a distraction due to conversation.

- **Exercise #4: Always sit down to eat your meal.**

When you go to eat, do so sitting down on a chair with your food on a table in front of you. This will help with digestion and help you to form a routine around eating. Try to avoid eating while standing up or walking as these create distractions. When you are physically up and about while eating, it will cause your mind to become distracted at the task at hand, as you will have to concentrate on your movement.

- **Exercise #5: Serve your meal on a plate or bowl.**

If possible, serve it on your favorite plate or bowl. Avoid eating food from the packet or take out containers as it makes eating feel less formal. This will help you pay more attention to your meal and its physical appearance.

- **Exercise #6: Make a conscious effort to chew your food thoroughly.**

Many people find themselves swallowing too soon and end up with digestion problems. Give your stomach an easier time with digesting by breaking down the food properly before swallowing.

- **Exercise #7: Make sure to eat only until you're 80% full.**

This is a fine line. Don't eat until you are certain you are full, but eat until you feel satisfied. A lot of the time, the feeling of fullness comes 10 minutes after you finish your meal. If you find yourself feeling full while you are still eating, you probably have overeaten.

- **Exercise #8: Take your time to truly savor the taste of food.**

Use all five of your senses. Before eating, take a look at your meal. Savor its look, smell, and overall appeal. Think about how each ingredient was cooked and seasoned and how you think the dish would taste because of it. During the meal, identify the taste of all the ingredients. What is the flavor? How does the flavor change if I eat different combinations of the ingredients? What can you smell? How does the texture feel in your mouth?

- **Exercise #9: Ask yourself how you feel about the food you are consuming.**

Do you feel happy? Pleasure? Guilt? Regret? Stress? Disappointment? Pay attention to the thoughts that the food brings to your mind. Does it bring up any memories? Fears? Beliefs? Give your food some serious consideration. How does your body feel after the meal compared to before? Do you feel energetic after eating, or do you feel lethargic? Does your stomach feel full or empty?

- **Exercise #10: Try to prepare your own meals where possible.**

The act of preparing food is proven to be psychologically beneficial and therapeutic. Make sure you are touching, tasting, and smelling the individual ingredients.

- **Exercise #11: Make a note of the difference in good food.**

This tends to be food that is fresh, seasonal, and minimally processed. Fresh and organic food tends to improve your overall mood and health. Food is our body's nourishment, and it provides the nutrition necessary for us to function optimally. Ingesting better quality food and ingredients is crucial to helping you feel better physically and psychologically.

How To Practice Mindful Eating

The key to mindful eating is to use all five of your senses. Doing this will bring your consciousness and your state of awareness into the present moment. This will also help you to avoid distractions. To practice mindful eating, try following along with the exercise below during your next meal, and try to do so every meal after that. Eventually, you will be able to practice this every time you eat.

Before you take a bite of your food, notice the smells of the food you are about to eat. Notice how it looks- the colors and textures. As you put food in your mouth, feel the textures of the food on your tongue. Notice all of the flavors that you are tasting and the feeling that they bring to your mouth. Notice how it feels when you chew the food- how it feels on your teeth and your cheeks. Doing this with every bite will bring you into the moment and ensure that you are consciously eating. Try practicing this with every meal.

Chapter 7: Intuitive Eating Meal Planning

Once you have come up with your general plan for your new lifestyle and how you want it to look, you can then begin planning more specifically. After you have gained an understanding of the principles of intuitive eating, you will be well equipped to begin this new style of eating.

What Is Meal Planning?

Planning your individual meals will make it much easier for you to reach for something nutritious and delicious when you are short on time. For example, when you get home from work or when you wake up tired in the morning and need to pack something for your lunch, you will not need to spend time planning your meals for the day.

You can plan your meals out a week in advance, two weeks or even a month if you wish. You can post this up on your fridge, and each day you will know exactly what you have ready to go, with no thinking required. When you do this, you will be able to step up to your fridge at dinner time and choose something that you want to eat you know you will provide your body with the nutrients it needs. You can heat it up in the oven and then begin to eat mindfully at the table.

By doing this preparation and planning in advance, you will allow yourself to benefit from eating healthy food and also the right proportion of food. Since you will have already planned out your meals, as well as each portion, you will take out the thinking, which will leave space for you to practice your mindful eating.

How Does Meal Planning Differ With Intuitive Eating Versus Dieting?

Regular meal planning involves looking at the week ahead and planning what you are going to eat based on the diet that you are following. For example, if you are on a Ketogenic diet, you would plan your meals with high-fat content and low carbohydrate content, and you would eat these meals during the week, regardless of what you feel like eating.

With intuitive meal planning, you will be able to plan your eating and thus, provide yourself with quick and easy meals that you can reheat or place in the oven in a pinch. This does not mean that you will stick to any specific diet plan. Rather, you will follow your intuitive eating principles to eat according to your body's signals. Having food prepared in advance will allow you to have fresh and healthy meals readily available to nourish your body. When you become hungry, you have healthy food right at your fingertips.

How To Meal Plan With Intuitive Eating

When it comes to meal planning with intuitive eating, you want to pre-prepare meals that will allow you to enjoy healthy and delicious options whenever you feel hungry. For this reason, you do not need to prepare specific meals to eat at specific times, but rather meals that you can reach for whenever you need them, knowing that you will enjoy the food. These meals will also be meals that you know will provide your body with the essential nutrients that it needs.

You can also prepare healthy snacks and treats that are actually good for you. There is nothing more rewarding than making your brain feel nourished while also replenishing your body. This can be as simple as a homemade trail mix with a bit of dark chocolate or a proportioned smoothie mix.

When you prepare food to eat for the week, try and add your favorite flavors to healthy food, and don't forget to keep it exciting with variety!

Chapter 8: Intuitive Eating Recipes

In this chapter, I will share with you some delicious recipes that you can try at home. These recipes are great for those who wish to try something new in the kitchen or who are becoming bored with their regular cycle of dinner meals.

Intuitive Eating Recipe Examples

Below are several recipes that you can try to make on your own at home so that you can feed your body new and delicious meals anytime!

Delicious Coconut Date Smoothie

Preparation Time: 5 Minutes
Cook Time: 1 Minute
Total Time: 6 Minutes

Ingredients:
- 2 cups almond milk or coconut milk
- 4 dates, (pitted)
- ¼ Cup spinach, frozen
- ¼ Cup chard, frozen (if possible)
- ¼ Cup kale, frozen (if possible)
- 1 cup strawberries, frozen
- 2 bananas
- 1 tbsp Chia seeds

- A small handful of ice cubes. You can adjust this amount depending on how many of your ingredients are frozen and how thick you want your smoothie to be.

Instructions
1. In your blender, add the almond milk, the dates, the spinach, kale, and the chard. We begin with only these

ingredients as they require extra blending because of all of their surface area.

2. Now, add in the strawberries, the two bananas, and the amount of ice that you have chosen. Blend until smooth

3. Pour into a large cup and add the chia seeds on top.

4. Serve and eat with a spoon or a straw

Egg And Avocado Rice Bowl

The first recipe we will look at is an Egg and Avocado Brown Rice Bowl. This recipe uses brown rice, garlic, and avocado, which are all good sources of Vitamin B6 or Pyridoxine. If you are a vegetarian, you can leave out the salmon, but if you add it, then you will be getting vitamin B1, or thiamine, as well as Omega-3 fatty acids. Further, the broccoli contains folic acid, and so does avocado. The egg used is also one that has been fortified with Omega-3.

Preparation Time: 10 Minutes
Cook Time: 40 Minutes
Total Time: 50 Minutes
Serves: 1

Ingredients:
- 1 Omega-3 Egg
- ¼ cup thinly sliced green onion
- Small bunch of broccoli
- Extra Virgin Olive Oil
- Half Avocado, sliced
- 1 Tsp Sesame Seeds
- 1 Tsp pickled ginger
- 1 Cup brown rice
- Salt and Pepper
- Splash Rice Wine Vinegar
- 1 salmon fillet

Instructions:
1. Bring your salmon out from the fridge so that it will be room temperature when you are ready to cook it.
2. Cook your brown rice according to its instructions. Feel free to make extra if you wish to expand this recipe into multiple portions or to save some for later to reheat.

3. If you are cooking the rice on the stovetop and you are unsure how you can follow the following instructions;

4. Put 1 cup of rinsed brown rice in a pot with 1 teaspoon of olive oil and 2 cups of water.
Bring the pot to a boil, then cover it and reduce the heat to low.
Simmer this pot of rice, water, and olive oil for 45 minutes.
Remove the rice from the burner and leave it to sit with its cover still on for approximately 10 minutes.
Fluff your rice with a fork to give it that loose texture.

5. With about twenty minutes left on your rice, preheat your oven to 400 degrees Fahrenheit. Cut your broccoli florets into small bite-size pieces and prepare your broccoli for roasting by placing the florets on a baking sheet and drizzle them with some olive oil. Sprinkle salt and pepper to taste. Toss them to spread the olive oil and the salt and pepper evenly. Place the baking sheet in the oven when it is preheated. Roast them in the oven until they are browned, and the stems are softened about fifteen minutes.

6. To cook your salmon, warm a non-stick pan on medium to low heat and place some drizzles of olive oil into the pan. Season your salmon as you wish with salt and pepper and then place it in the pan with the skin facing up. Cook for about four minutes, or until it is golden brown, and then flip it. On this second side, cook it until it is firm when you press into it, and the skin becomes crispy. This second side will take roughly three minutes.

7. When your rice and your broccoli is almost finished, fry your egg in a pan with a bit of olive oil until it is cooked through.

8. You can either remove the skin from your salmon or leave it on, whichever you wish.

9. When your broccoli is ready, place it on your rice bowl along with your salmon. Then add your fried egg, your sliced

avocado, your sliced green onion, pickled ginger, and finally, the sesame seeds. Add a splash of rice wine vinegar to the bowl and you are ready to eat.

Breakfast Oats

A great breakfast recipe and one that you can prepare in a very short amount of time. Whole grain oats contain iron, and if you add fruits to it like bananas and raspberries, these contain magnesium. The apricots will give the oats sweetness without sugar and also contain iron. Adding nuts like almonds will give you protein and adding milk or yogurt as well will add calcium to your diet.

Preparation Time: 5 Minutes
Cook Time: 5 Minutes
Total time: 5 Minutes

Serves 1
Ingredients:
- ¾ Cup plain Whole grain oats
- ¼ cup almonds, sliced
- ½ Banana, sliced
- ¼ Cup raspberries
- ¾ Cup cinnamon, ground
- ¼ Cup dried apricots

Instructions:
1. Add the oats and 1 ½ cups of water to a small pot. Turn on the burner to high heat and bring these ingredients up to a boil. When this occurs, turn the heat down to medium to low and let it cook for five minutes, or until there is no water left unabsorbed.
2. Remove this from the heat and then transfer the cooked oats to a bowl.
3. Pour in the cinnamon, the almonds, bananas, apricots, and raspberries in whatever order you wish.
4. Eat it while still hot for best taste

Braised Chicken On A Bed Of Lentils And Mushrooms

This recipe contains chicken thighs which are an excellent source of vitamin K2, as well as lentils which will provide you with your calcium and mushrooms which are the only plant source that naturally contains Vitamin D. This recipe is a triple threat when it comes to your health, and it tastes great to boot!

Preparation Time: 10 Minutes
Cook Time: 35 Minutes
Total Time: 45 Minutes

Serves 4
Ingredients:

- 4 chicken thighs
- 1 onion
- 2 Cups Mushrooms of your choice (400g)
- 2 Cups lentils (green or any of your choice)
- 2 cloves of garlic, diced
- 2 Tbsp olive oil
- 2.5 cups water
- 1 tsp salt
- Black pepper grinder
- ⅔ Cup chicken broth (low sodium)
- 2 tbsp parsley, chopped
- 2 tbsp lemon juice

Instructions:
1. In a large pot, add the lentils and the water as well as ¾ of the tsp of salt. Bring this to a boil on high heat.
2. Once boiling, bring the heat down to low to medium heat and let the lentils simmer with a lid covering the pot for 25 minutes. You want the lentils to be soft but not breaking into pieces.

3. While the lentils are cooking, get a large pan and place 1 tbsp of olive oil in it. Add the onion, the garlic, and the mushrooms. Cook this on low heat until the onions turn clear and are aromatic.

4. When the lentils are done, add the mixture of onions, garlic, and mushrooms to the lentils in the pot.

5. Add 1 tbsp of oil in the now-empty pan on medium heat.

6. While you are doing this, use ¼ teaspoon of salt and some black pepper and put the chicken into the heated pan.

7. Cook the chicken until it becomes browned. This will take roughly 12 minutes.

8. Pour the remaining oil and any fat out of the pan and into a small bowl. Don't throw this out yet.

9. Add your chicken broth to the pan with chicken and then bring the heat down to low and put a lid on the pan before letting it simmer for 15 minutes.

10. Add the juice and fat that you put aside earlier to the pit of lentils and vegetables.

11. Add as well the chopped parsley and some lemon juice to the pot of lentils and vegetables.

12. Add the now cooked chicken into the lentils pot and put the lid on. Let this sit for 5 minutes.

13. After the 5 minutes have passed, you are ready to eat!

14. Garnish with salt and pepper if you wish, plate, and serve.

Beef And Broccoli Stir-Fry

Preparation Time: 16 minutes
Cooking time: 12 minutes
Total Time: 28 minutes

Makes: 4 Servings
Serving Size: 1 and ¼ of a cup or ¼ of total recipe

Ingredients:
- Sirloin Beef, Lean and thinly sliced- ¾ of a pound
- Cornstarch- 2 and 1/3 tablespoons
- Red pepper flakes- 2 tablespoons
- Chicken Broth, Reduced Sodium- 1 Cup
- Salt- ¼ teaspoon
- Broccoli- 5 cups
- Water- ¼ cup
- Ginger root, minced- 1 tablespoon
- Garlic, minced- 2 tablespoons
- Soy Sauce, low sodium- ¼ cup

Instructions:
1. Take a large plate and spread the cornstarch and the salt around the plate evenly. Take the beef strips and coat them with the mixture.
2. Using a wok or a deep pan, put the oil in and heat it up on the medium to high heat level
3. Put the beef in when the pan is hot and cook this until it is cooked all the way through- you will know as it will turn brown. This will take about 4 minutes.
4. Use a slotted spoon and take the beef out of the pan and place it on a new plate.
5. In the same pan with the heated oil and the beef drippings, put ½ cup of reduced-sodium chicken broth. Begin stirring this in the pan to combine everything and loosen the residue on the pan.

6. Put the broccoli in the pan and cook it with the lid on. Add some water if you need it.
7. When the broccoli is becoming softer but not fully cooked yet-this will take about 3 minutes, take the lid off and put the garlic, ginger, and red pepper flakes in. Fry this until it becomes noticeably fragrant, which will take roughly one minute.
8. Using a vessel of your choice, mix the rest of the broth (1/2 cup), the soy sauce, the water, and the rest of the cornstarch (1/2 tablespoon). Stir it to mix well.
9. Put this sauce mix into the wok and stir everything to combine it all.
10. Bring the heat down to a medium to low level and let this simmer.
11. Simmer for about a minute, until it begins to become thicker.
12. Put the beef in the pan once again and stir everything, so the beef becomes coated.
13. It is now ready to serve!

Intuitive Eating With Food Allergies Or Restrictions

You may be wondering, at this point in the book, what you should do, or if it is even possible for you to practice intuitive eating if you have allergies or food restrictions. The answer to this question is a resounding "Yes". No matter your allergies or dietary restrictions, it is possible to practice intuitive eating.

Since intuitive eating aims to help you get back to your body's natural state of being, where you follow its desires and needs, you can practice this no matter what foods you normally eat. Whether you are a vegetarian, a vegan, have celiac disease, are allergic to peanuts or anything else, you can still listen to your body, follow the nine rules of intuitive eating and get back to your body's preferred method of eating.

Tips For Intuitive Eating With Food Allergies Or Restrictions

• Listen to your body

While you cannot give in to every craving or every desire that your body has, you can still listen to your body when it comes to intuitive eating with allergies or dietary restrictions. You can listen to when your body is hungry, what your body needs to eat or drink, or how much it needs to eat.

• Adhere to your restrictions or allergies

Just because you are practicing intuitive eating does not mean that you need to give into every type of food item that you feel like eating. You can still maintain your prescribed diet while practicing intuitive eating, while avoiding the foods you are allergic to. As long as you keep this in mind, all of the other rules of intuitive eating still apply.

Intuitive Eating Recipes For Food Allergies Or Restrictions

Below you can find recipes that will help you to make delicious and healthy foods while still adhering to your dietary restrictions or allergies.

Fresh Green Beans with Tofu And Mushroom Stir-Fry

If you are a vegetarian, this recipe is a great option for a quick and delicious dinner that does not include meat, and that instead includes tofu as a great protein source.

Nutritional Information:
Serving: 1 Serving (1/6 of Recipe)
Calories: 94kcal
Carbohydrates: 9g
Protein: 5g
Fat: 5g
Saturated Fat: 2g
Fiber: 3g
Sugar: 4g

15 minutes: Prep Time
20 minutes: Cook Time
35 minutes: Total Time

Servings: 6 Servings

Ingredients:
- 1/4 teaspoon kosher salt
- 1-pound thin green beans trimmed
- 1 cup tofu, firm variety
- 1 tablespoon minced fresh sage
- 1 large shallot minced
- 12 ounces mushrooms thinly sliced

- 1 teaspoon olive oil
- 3 tablespoons parsley minced
- 1 tablespoon minced fresh thyme leaves
- 1/4 teaspoon freshly ground black pepper
- 1 tablespoon ginger, grated
- 1 tablespoon soy sauce

Instructions:

1. Salt a large saucepan full of water and heat it up until it boils. Mix your beans into the water and cook them until they become tender but still a little crispy, this will take approximately 2 minutes. Drain the water and immediately move the cooked beans to a bowl full of ice and water to stop them from cooking any further.
2. Drain the beans of the water once again and set them aside.
3. Put your tofu inside of a big frying pan on one-half level of heat. Heat your tofu until it becomes crispy. Move the tofu to a paper towel and crumble it with your hands before setting it off to the side for later.
4. Put olive oil into the same frying pan you used before and turn it on to medium-high heat. Add in your mushrooms and shallots, and cook them until they are tender, this will take approx—2 to 3 minutes.
5. Add the green beans to the frying pan again and cook the entire thing for 1 to 2 minutes more, stir it often.
6. Add in the sage, thyme, parsley, pepper and, salt, and stir it to combine. Cook this for another minute, before re-adding your tofu.
7. Serve this dish either hot or at room temperature.

Vegan Chana Masala Curry

If you are vegan, this is a delicious and healthy curry recipe that you can make that also adheres to your diet restrictions.

Nutritional Information:
Calories: 371
Calories from Fat: 88
Total Fat: 10g
Carbohydrates: 59 grams
Protein: 17 grams

Servings: Makes 4 Servings

Ingredients:
- Olive Oil-1 Tablespoon
- Cayenne Pepper- 1/8 of a tablespoon
- Diced Tomatoes- 28 ounces diced
- Garam Masala- 2 tablespoons
- Jalapeno Pepper- 1
- Onion- 1 diced
- Ginger- 1 tablespoon shaved
- Garlic- 4 cloves minced
- Chickpeas- canned- 28 ounces (be sure to drain the liquid and rinse them before using them in the recipe)

Instructions:
1. Take a big wok and put the olive oil into it
2. Once heated, add in your onions and sauté them until they are sweating and softened. This will take about 5 minutes.
3. Add in your ginger, jalapeno, and your garlic, and then cook this mixture for another minute
4. Sprinkle in your spices (pepper, salt, coriander, turmeric, garam masala, cumin, cayenne pepper). Then, cook this for another minute. The mixture will become fragrant as you do this.
5. Add your chickpeas and tomatoes into the fragrant mixture in the wok. Let this simmer.

6. Cover the pan and let this simmer for about twenty minutes.
7. After it simmers for the allotted time, give it a taste test and season it if you feel it could be spicier or if it needs more salt. You might want to mix in some more of the garam masala if you want it to be stronger in flavor.
8. Serve and enjoy this meal that is only 1 Smart Point per serving!

Chapter 9: Intuitive Eating While Pregnant

You may have heard of the whacky cravings that many women experience during pregnancy. With the onset of the second trimester come these very strong cravings that nobody can truly understand but the pregnant woman who is needing ice cream with pickles right away! The second trimester is when these cravings will be at an all-time high. You may also experience some aversions to certain foods at the same time as your cravings begin around the end of the first and beginning of the second trimester.

You may wonder "when it is okay to give in to these cravings"? Some of them may be for things that are not wildly unhealthy, like a sandwich with lots of mustard or some sweet things like fruits mixed in with pudding. These cravings are okay to give in to from time to time, especially if they are fleeting. You must ensure, however, that the majority of your meals are balanced and healthy, giving both you and your baby the nutrients you need.

Craving Examples And Substitutions

- Carbohydrates

If you crave foods like carbohydrates, try to combine them with a protein. An example of this is cheese and crackers. This is a healthier snack than crackers alone.

- Fast Foods

If you are feeling a lot of cravings that are for candies, chips, fast-foods and other objectively unhealthy foods most of the time, it will not be beneficial to you and your baby to eat these foods every day. Supplements can sometimes help with a situation like this, where you will be craving certain foods and unable to stomach others. Supplements can help you to get the vitamins and nutrients that you need if you cannot get them from real foods. Your first option, however, should always be natural food.

- Caffeine

Another craving that will likely be nagging at you during the beginning of your pregnancy is the craving for caffeine. It is always important to watch your caffeine intake during pregnancy.

Caffeine is okay in very small amounts, but it should not be consumed at high levels. This is especially important in the first trimester because of the potential of miscarriage that it can cause. Caffeine consumption during pregnancy has also been shown to lead to premature delivery as well as low birth weight. In some cases, a baby can even exhibit withdrawal symptoms from caffeine. To be safe, it is better to avoid caffeine, especially in the first trimester.

Caffeine also dehydrates the consumer, so it is essential to ensure you are properly hydrated if you are consuming any caffeine. Instead of coffee, try drinking an herbal tea or flavored water to give yourself a pleasant drink to sip on.

Foods To Avoid

While you can certainly follow intuitive eating during pregnancy, some foods should be avoided when pregnant. Though intuitive eating does not involve any kind of restriction or diet mentality, it is important to ensure that you are keeping both yourself and your baby safe. In this section, we will look at the foods that you should not eat while pregnant.

- Listeria

Deli meats can sometimes contain Listeria, which is a bacteria that is not as serious to adults on our own, but if you are pregnant, this can be very damaging to your unborn baby. The reason why listeria is so damaging is that it can reach the baby through the placenta and can poison the baby's blood or give it an infection, which could potentially lead to a miscarriage.

Smoked Foods should be avoided for the same reason as deli meats, as these can contain listeria as well. These foods include smoked fish, (like lox) as well as meat jerky.

Soft Cheeses like blue cheese, feta, and queso should be avoided because they can also contain listeria. The unpasteurized milk used to make this cheese is what makes them potentially harmful. Though, if the soft cheese is not imported, and if it is made with pasteurized milk, it is likely safe.

- Tuna

While tuna doesn't need to be avoided altogether, canned tuna should be consumed at a minimum as well as other fish such as mackerel and swordfish. These types of fish are known to contain mercury at higher levels than others. Mercury can be harmful to your baby by causing brain development issues or brain damage, so be sure to avoid these. Especially during the first trimester when everything in the baby's body is rapidly forming. Be careful when eating sushi as sometimes the fish used in sushi can contain mercury in high amounts.

- Salmonella

Salmonella is harmful to humans if they become infected, but it is even more harmful to unborn babies. Salmonella can infect the fluid that surrounds the baby in the placenta, which can then lead to a miscarriage. Salmonella poisoning can cause the mother to become quite sick, which is not ideal for a woman who is carrying a growing baby. This is because all of her resources need to go towards helping the baby to grow into a strong and healthy individual.

To avoid risking exposure to salmonella, **raw eggs,** and anything containing raw eggs should be avoided altogether. Some dressings and sauces can contain raw eggs, and so you should be careful when consuming these. Further, **raw meats** can contain salmonellae such as chicken, turkey, **raw seafood,** and rare beef such as steaks.

Avoid eating uncooked clams, oysters, eggs, and meats like a rare steak. This can leave you at risk of different foodborne pathogens that can harm your baby.

In the third trimester, you should avoid the same things as you should avoid in the first and second trimesters like smoked fish and meats, deli meats, uncooked eggs, raw meats, and caffeine. There are some additional things to avoid as well in this trimester, though, which are listed below for you.

- Cat litter

You should avoid cat litter as it can contain a parasite that has been known to lead to toxoplasmosis. This can also be contracted through **undercooked meat**. This disease can be transmitted to your baby if you are infected with it, which is why it should be heavily prevented. This disease can give flu-like symptoms, which to an adult may not be so bad, but to an unborn baby, this could be detrimental.

- Uncooked sprouts

Uncooked sprouts should also be avoided. Bacteria like those we discussed in the previous chapters- listeria and salmonella in addition to E.coli, can be found in sprouts because of the cracks in their shells. So, if you want to eat them, you must thoroughly cook them first to kill any bacteria that maybe there.

- Raw fish

Raw fish should be avoided. This is because it contains mercury, which is unhealthy for your unborn baby. Cooked fish are safe to eat, but only eeaten in moderate quantities- no more than twice per week.

Intuitive Eating Post-Pregnancy

After giving birth, it is important to take some time to rest and recuperate. Beginning a strict diet immediately after giving birth in an attempt to lose extra weight, is not a good idea. This is because a weight loss diet will reduce the quality of breast milk that your body produces.

Believe it or not, performing the act of breastfeeding each day causes you to burn calories. Just like when you were still pregnant, you will still need to consume more calories than you regularly would have before you became pregnant. For this reason, don't go on any sort of diet while breastfeeding, and don't begin to watch what you eat unless it is to ensure you are eating enough of the nutrients that you and your baby need. You will want to have as many nutrients and calories as your baby requires, so listen to your hunger and follow what it is telling you, especially while breastfeeding.

Caffeine Post-Pregnancy

If you were a regular coffee drinker before you became pregnant, you will likely be looking for the coffee pot after giving birth.

The problem is, it is important to watch your caffeine consumption while breastfeeding. Caffeine has been shown to affect breastmilk, and therefore, the baby as well. Having too much caffeine as a breastfeeding mother can lead to your baby receiving it through the milk and, in turn, becoming fussy and extra energetic afterward. You also want to avoid having your baby become dependent on caffeine, as this is not healthy. Caffeine can also lead to dehydration, and the last thing you want is a dehydrated baby. You can have some caffeine, but no more than 24 ounces per day, preferably in 3 different 8-ounce servings and no more than this.

Bonus: How to Teach Your Child Mindful Eating

Since our childhood and developmental history play a big role in who we are today, it is important to raise your child in an intentional way, instilling habits and beliefs that will benefit them early on. In this chapter, we will look at how you can raise a mindful eater and a child who practices intuitive eating.

How To Transform Your Child's Relationship With Food

In this section, we are going to discuss several ways that you can help your child to develop a healthy relationship with food.

- Avoid using food as a reward

If you teach your child that food is used as a reward, it can lead them away from intuitive eating and towards an unhealthy relationship with food.

- Avoid using food as a punishment

Similar to how using food as a reward can lead your child to develop an unhealthy relationship with food, using food as a punishment t can lead your child to develop an unhealthy relationship with food. Examples of this include withholding food or not allowing certain foods as a form of punishment.

- Set a good example

Food can be seen as something that you need to survive, as a form of stress-relief through the enjoyment of cooking healthy foods and as a way to bring people together. By viewing food and food preparation in this way, you can shift your perspective and change your relationship with food. By doing this within your own life, you can impart this wisdom on your child and help them develop into a little human with a healthy relationship to food.

How To Encourage Your Child To Practice Intuitive Eating

To help your child become an intuitive eater, one of the greatest things that you can do is model this type of behavior for them. Using the information in this chapter, you will be able to help your child have a better relationship with food. This will also help you to develop your child into an intuitive eater.

For the most part, children are already much better equipped to become successful intuitive eaters, as they have not been exposed to the diet culture and all of the shame and punishment that comes with it. For this reason, teaching them about intuitive eating will likely be much easier and require much less work than teaching yourself or other adults.

Children are usually better able to practice mindfulness than adults can, as they are likely get in touch with the sensations and feelings of their body with much more ease than adults can. By encouraging them and reminding them that they should listen to their body, they will not be as affected by the media and the diet culture that will eventually make its way into their view.

How To Encourage Your Child To Practice Mindful Eating

We have discussed mindfulness several times throughout this book, and here we are going to discuss how you can encourage your child to become a mindful eater.

Mindfulness is not a practice that is reserved only for adults; mindfulness is a technique that can be performed by children as well. Mindfulness can help children to fine-tune their mind-body connection. One great way to do this is to help your child perform the body scan meditation, as you learned in the "listen to your body" section of this book. This practice will help them to identify what they are feeling physically and mentally, and where they are feeling it as well. By helping your child to practice this kind of mindfulness, you will introduce them to the idea of mindfulness, and you can then incorporate it into their eating practices. Once you get them acquainted with their bodies from the inside out, doing this while sitting at the table for a meal will be much easier for them.

Further, scientific research points to the conclusion that there are numerous physical and psychological benefits to relieving tension and relaxing your body, even for children. The body scan meditation is a very effective and useful meditation technique that can help both you and your child to stay physically and mentally relaxed. It can help you return to a calm state when you notice that your child is not being mindful at the dinner table. This could be caused by a large number of distractions, for example. Here is a guide on how you can try the body scan meditation. You may wish to try this on your own first, and then try it with your child by reading out the directions to them and helping them if they have any questions.

In no time, your child will be able to do an abbreviated version of this meditation by sitting down and bringing awareness to any place in your body where you feel that you are carrying tension. This can then translate to the dinner table, where they can bring attention and awareness to their mouth and eating food.

Another great way to help your child practice mindfulness is by walking them through a basic mindfulness meditation that is great for beginners. Begin by reading the following instructions aloud to them in a low and soft voice, encouraging relaxation and attention to their body. Remind them of the benefits that mindful eating can provide them with, such as better digestion, better relaxation, and overall healthier eating habits.

1. Find a quiet place that you feel comfortable in—ideally, your home or someone where you feel safe. Sit in a chair or on the floor. Make sure your head and back are straight but are not tense.
2. Try to sort your thoughts and put aside those that are of the past and future. Stick to the thoughts about the present.
3. Bring your awareness to your breath. Make sure to focus on the feeling and sensation of air moving through your body as you inhale and exhale. Feel the way your belly rises and falls. Feel the air enter through your nostrils and leave through your mouth. Make sure to pay attention to the differences in each breath.
4. Watch every thought come and go. Act as if you are watching the clouds, letting them pass by you as you watch each one. Whether your thought is a worry, fear, anxiety, or hope - when these thoughts come up, don't ignore them or try to suppress them. Simply acknowledge them, remain calm, and anchor yourself with your breathing.
5. You may find yourself getting carried away in your thoughts. If this happens, observe where your mind wandered, and without passing judgment on yourself, return focus to your breaths. Keep in mind that this happens a lot with beginners; try not to be too hard on yourself when this occurs. Always use your breathing as an anchor again.
6. As we near the end of the session, sit for a minute or two and become aware of where you physically are. Get up gradually.

By helping your child to practice this type of mindfulness meditation, you will be able to encourage them to use this practice when they are at the dinner table. Eventually, your entire family will be able to practice mindful eating at the table together and experience the joys that intuitive eating can bring to your life.

Intuitive Eating Quick Tips

Before this book concludes, I want to leave you with a few more tips to stay on course with intuitive eating.

- Tip 1: Self-Evaluate

Before you begin, take some time to look at your existing eating habits, patterns, and behaviors and analyze them.

- Tip 2: Self-Rank

When you finish eating a meal, rank your level of fullness on a scale of 1 to 10, 1 being extremely hungry and 10 being extremely stuffed. This will help you to determine if you are successfully stopping when you are satisfied and not overeating.

- Tip 3: Listen

As you know by now, listening to your body, your emotions and your mind is extremely important when it comes to intuitive eating. As long as you remember this, you will be well on your way to becoming a lifelong intuitive eater.

- Tip 4: Keep Practicing

If you have learned anything in this book, it is that you should allow yourself the space to learn and grow. Making mistakes is part of the journey. You should allow yourself to learn as you go and do not expect perfection right away. If you are dedicated to becoming an intuitive eater, you should allow yourself the time to practice. Just like any skill, you will need to practice and develop your skills of listening to your body and giving it what it needs.

- Tip 5: Maintain a "Growth Mindset"

Success depends on whether or not a person has a growth mindset. A fixed mindset is when a person believes that their intelligence and skills are a fixed trait (O'Brien 2018). They have what they have, and that's it. This makes the person highly concerned with what skills and intelligence they currently have, and they do not focus on what they can gain. Therefore, their activities are limited to the capacity that they think they have. However, those with growth mindsets understand that any skill can be developed and improved upon throughout their life.

This can be done through education, training, or simply just even passion. They understand that their brain is a muscle that can be 'worked out' to grow stronger. Knowing this, you must employ a growth mindset. Every single skill you have can be ameliorated by putting in the effort to see it from a growth mindset. This is the mindset for success when it comes to life in general, but especially when it comes to changing something about your lifestyle- like learning to practice intuitive eating.

Conclusion

You began this book as someone who was unable to stop disordered overeating and who was unsure of where to turn for support and advice. Now, you have found the solution to this problem and have learned everything you need to know about the "non-diet method of intuitive eating." In this book, we discussed intuitive eating and intuitive movement at-length. Now you are equipped with a solution once and for all! This method has been proven to work for many people. You are now ready to put this into practice, where you will find yourself with a new lease on life.

In this book, we discussed what intuitive eating is and the science behind why it works. We also discussed the benefits that you will find through following an intuitive eating style, and we looked at the nine rules of intuitive eating, which include the following:

1. Adhere to your hunger
2. Say no to the diet industry
3. Don't restrict what you eat
4. Recognize when you are full
5. Eliminate dietary thinking
6. Don't eat out of "emotional hunger."
7. Don't self-judge
8. Exercise using intuitive movement
9. Listen to your body

In addition to these principles, we also looked at what emotional eating is and how you can make peace with your body. You learned how to properly compose your plate of food, develop a meal plan and engage in mindful eating. You were also given several nutritious recipes that you can try at home.

Finally, we looked at some tips for intuitive eating for women who are pregnant and for parents who wish to raise their children as mindful eaters. All of these topics and more made for a book packed with valuable information that will be available to you any time you need it.

As you begin your journey of intuitive eating, you will find that you develop a higher level of self-esteem, along with, better feelings about your body image. You find that you have more optimism about life in general. You also have numerous health benefits including a lower body mass index, higher HDL cholesterol levels and lower triglyceride levels. Emotional and disordered eating finally becomes less frequent. With all this being said, you are well on your way to becoming the best version of yourself.

The one major takeaway that I want you to get through reading this book is a new perspective on dieting and eating well. I also want you to walk away with a new perspective on exercise and movement of your body. With these new ways of viewing your body and yourself, I want you to leave this book with a new sense of self and a new lease on life. You have taken your health into your own hands, and you are now able to see that you don't have to force yourself to follow a diet that is doomed from the start or an exercise plan that does not fit with your body or your mind. If you can understand this, you have gained the most valuable piece of information that this book has to offer you. Today is the best today to start improving your health. Good luck on your journey!

References

"Body Scan Meditation" (2019, April 16). Retrieved from https://www.igrc.org/blogpostsdetail/body-scan-meditation-12794843

Agrawal, A. (2019, June 20). *Mindfulness Meditation – What It Is And How To Do It.* Inspired Journey towards greater heights -learnings and sharing. Retrieved from https://befinexpert.wordpress.com/2019/06/20/mindfulness-meditation-what-it-is-and-how-to-do-it

Beech, S. (2019). *Mindful Eating.* The Psych Professionals. Retrieved from https://psychprofessionals.com.au/mindful-eating

O'Brien, D. (2018, August 1). *Back to School With a Growth Mindset.* Dynamath. Retrieved from https://dynamath.scholastic.com/pages/dynamath-expressions/2018-19/back-to-school-with-a-growth-mindset.html

Printed in Great Britain
by Amazon